A Quick Reference to
MEDICAL TERMINOLOGY

A Quick Reference to
MEDICAL TERMINOLOGY

Juanita J. Davies

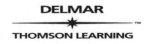

DELMAR

THOMSON LEARNING

Australia   Canada   Mexico   Singapore   Spain   United Kingdom   United States

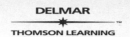

DELMAR
THOMSON LEARNING ™

A Quick Reference to Medical Terminology
by Juanita J. Davies

Health Care Publishing Director: William Brottmiller
Executive Editor: Cathy L. Esperti
Acquisitions Editor: Sherry Gomoll
Executive Marketing Manager: Dawn F. Gerrain
Channel Manager: Jennifer McAvey
Editorial Assistant: Jennifer Conklin
Art/Design Coordinator: Connie Lundberg-Watkins
Project Editor: David Buddle
Production Coordinator: Anne Sherman

Printed in Canada
1 2 3 4 5 XXX 06 05 04 03 02

For more information, contact Delmar Learning,
5 Maxwell Drive
Clifton Park, NY 1065
Or find us on the World Wide Web at http://www.delmar.com

Library of Congress Cataloging-in-Publication Data
Davies, Juanita J.
    A quick reference to medical terminology / by Juanita Davies.
        p.   cm
    ISBN 0-7668-4060-3
    1. Medicine—Terminology—Handbooks, manuals, etc.   I. Title.
R123 .D284 2002
610'.1'4—dc21

                        2001047830

NOTICE TO THE READER

To my students

Contents

Appendices

**Index to Labeled Structures
Found in Figures** 307

Preface

WHO THIS BOOK IS FOR

This handbook was created specifically for students, teachers, and allied health professionals who want an inexpensive and succinct teaching, and reference text for medical terminology.

Students taking any allied health program or an individual course in anatomy, physiology, or pathology will have to learn medical language. This is not so easy. Medical words can be overwhelming. They are not part of everyday English, and can be long and complex (*laryngotracheobronchitis*!). There are so many, how is a student supposed to remember them all? This book can help—*a lot*. It is filled with definitions of medical words encountered in such courses. It has an appendix that teaches the student, in very simplified form, how medical words are formed, so that the process of learning them and figuring out the probable meaning of a new term is made easy. Additionally, handy devices called *Memory Keys* help the student remember the parts of medical terms and provide interesting facts about their derivation.

Professionals in every branch of medical practice will find this book to be a highly portable, accurate, and handy reference. Teachers of an introductory course will enjoy these benefits, along with the special features added specifically to assist their students in learning terminology.

WHAT THE BOOK CONTAINS

1. **Term Definitions.** The first part of the book contains a list of the most common medical terms listed under the relevant prefix, root, or suffix, except when the term cannot be broken down into component parts. Each term is defined in simple and easy-to-understand language, and Memory Keys are sprinkled throughout to aid learning and to add interest.
2. **Term Analysis.** Appendix A briefly outlines the system used for learning medical language, which can be particularly useful for students and a good refresher for working professionals. Students who take a little time to study this part

of the book at the beginning of their course, will find it much easier to acquire an extensive medical vocabulary because they will not have to merely memorize. Instead, they will be able to figure out meanings for themselves because they will know how to analyze terms. By studying the most common word elements used in medical words, students will be able to define unfamiliar medical terms when they are encountered, and in no time will find their medical vocabulary greatly expanded. This easy-to-learn system involves:

- Analyzing medical words into their word elements (prefixes, roots, or suffixes)
- Defining the word elements, which results in defining the medical word
- Learning to combine and recombine the word elements into medical words

3. **Pronunciation.** Appendix B contains a simple guide to common pronunciation.
4. **Plural Formation.** Appendix C sets out the rules for forming plurals.
5. **Suffixes.** Appendix D contains a list of common suffixes.
6. **Prefixes.** Appendix E contains a list of common prefixes.
7. **Illustrations of Body Systems.** Appendix F rounds out the book as both a terminology text and reference book by providing illustrations for all the body systems, so that students and professionals alike have ready reference to pictorial context for the terms contained in the book.

HOW TO LOOK UP A TERM

Since the book is not a dictionary, it is not organized like one. Those terms that cannot be broken down into component parts are listed in strict alphabetical order, but the rest are grouped under a common prefix, root, or suffix that is listed in alphabetical order. Thus, unlike a dictionary, *anemia* is found before the term *abductor*, because *anemia* is listed under the prefix *a-*, while *abductor* is listed under the prefix *ab-*, which of course comes later. This grouping or chunking of terms under the same word element reinforces the method of analyzing terms described in Appendix A, and therefore makes terms easier for students to learn and remember. A little effort and study will enable students to readily find them. The professional who knows how to analyze terms will have no trouble.

This approach to a reference text requires that a fair bit of redundancy be built into the structure of the book, and thus some entries are repeated. For example, *diagnosis* is defined under the prefix *dia-* and under the suffix *-gnosis*. This is advantageous to the student learning terminology, and is convenient to the professional using the book as a reference. In the majority of cases, the more complete definition is found in the entry appearing under the first letter of the word. A simpler definition is found under the suffix, together with a reference to the more extensive definition.

ACKNOWLEDGMENTS

I wish to thank the editors of Delmar Learning, especially Cathy Esperti, Executive Editor, whose timely advice gave shape to this project; Dave Buddle, Project Editor, whose thoroughness and diligence enhanced the quality of the text; and the production staff of Delmar who worked hard to bring this book to publication.

I must mention too, the help given to me by my husband Jim Davies, who over a two-year period, helped immeasurably by working countless hours reading, editing, and providing wise counsel.

Listing of Medical Terms and Word Elements

a- no; not; lack of

Memory Key: **a-** changes to **an-** before word elements beginning with a vowel.

achalasia inability of the muscles of the digestive tract to relax

achlorhydria lack of hydrochloric acid

achondroplasia lack of cartilage formation leading to a type of dwarfism

afebrile no fever

agranulocyte a type of leukocyte characterized by the lack of granules within the cell membrane. Examples: lymphocytes and monocytes.

agranulocytosis abnormal condition characterized by a lack of granulocytes

akinesia lack of movement

amenorrhea no menstruation

amnesia pathological loss of memory

anaerobic oxygen is not required for survival

analgesia not feeling any pain

Memory Key: Tylenol is an analgesic drug used to relieve pain.

anemia lack of red blood cells or hemoglobin. Examples include:

   iron deficiency a.: anemia caused by inadequate iron absorption or increased iron requirements

   pernicious a.: reduction of red blood cells due to the lack of vitamin B_{12}

   sickle-cell a.: genetic hemolytic anemia in which red blood cells assume sickle shapes rather than biconcave discs. Once the red blood cells sickle, they become rigid, obstructing blood flow.

anencephaly congenital absence of the brain

anesthesia loss of sensation or ability to feel pain caused by injury or the administration of a drug

anhidrosis lack of sweat

anisocytosis increased variation in the size of red blood cells

anomaly an abnormality; deviation from the norm

anorchia congenital absence of one or both testicles

anorexia loss of appetite often accompanying a feeling of sickness

anorexia nervosa loss of appetite leading to extreme thinness; caused by underlying psychological problems

anovulation no ovulation

anoxia lack or deficiency of oxygen; may be used interchangeably with *hypoxia*

aspermatogenesis no sperm formation

anuria no urine formation; suppression

apathy lack of feeling or emotions

Memory Key: The suffix **-pathy** comes from the Greek word *pathos* which means "deep emotion." It wasn't until some time later that **-pathy** was used to mean "disease."

aphakia absence of the lens of the eye

aphasia loss or impairment of speech

aphonia loss of voice; hoarseness

apnea no breathing

apraxia inability to perform purposeful movements in the absence of paralysis. For example, an apraxic patient may not be able to swing a baseball bat despite being repeatedly shown the movements.

arrhythmia deviations from the normal heart rhythm

Memory Key: An- changes to **ar-** before roots starting with **r**.

aseptic free from infectious material

asphyxia no pulse

asthenia without strength

astigmatism an error of refraction due to defective curvature of the cornea or lens of the eye, preventing light rays from focussing on the same point on the retina, thus causing impaired vision. **Stigmat/o** means "point."

ataxia lack of muscle coordination

atony lack of muscle tone

atresia no opening

atrophy wasting away or decrease in size of cells, tissues, or organs

Memory Key: When a muscle is not used it gets smaller. For example, when a plaster of Paris cast is removed from a limb, the muscles will be noticeably smaller because they have not been used. The muscles have **atrophied**.

avascular no blood vessels

ab- away from

abduct to draw away

abduction the process of drawing a part, such as the arm or leg, away from the midline of the body

abductor that which draws away from the midline of the body. For example, the abductor muscles draw the thigh away from the midline.

aberrant deviation from the normal course

abortion premature expulsion of the products of conception

spontaneous a.: naturally occurring abortion. Also called a miscarriage.

therapeutic a.: abortion performed to save the life or health (mental or physical) of the pregnant woman.

abrasion a scraping away of skin, often due to trauma. The word element **ras** means "to scrape."

Memory Key: A man can use a razor to scrape off his beard.

abruptio placenta premature separation of the placenta

abscess a pus-filled cavity in tissues and organs

Memory Key: In ancient Roman medicine, it was thought that pus was bad fluid thrown *away from* the body.

absorption the passing substances into body tissues or fluids

abd- hide

*abd*omen the area of the body between the thorax and pelvis containing a cavity or hollow space in which body organs are hidden

Memory Key: Do not confuse abdomen with stomach. The stomach is an organ within the abdomen.

abdomin/o abdomen

*abdomin*al pertaining to the abdomen

Memory Key: The English word *abdomen* is spelled with an **e**, but the medical root abdomin/o is spelled with an **i**.

*abdomin*al reflex. See **reflex**.

*abdomin*ocentesis surgical puncture of the peritoneal cavity to remove fluid. Also known as *paracentesis*.

*abdomin*opelvic pertaining to the abdomen and pelvis

absence seizure See seizure.

ac- sharp; pointed

*ac*ute an acute disease is of sharp or sudden onset, of short duration, and is severe. Compare with **chronic** and **subacute**.

acanth/o thorny; spiny

*acanth*olysis breakdown or separation of the prickle-cell layer of the epidermis leading to cellular degeneration

Memory Key I: Acanth/o literally means a "pointy flower"; its reference is to a prickly or thorny plant featured in ancient Greek architecture.

Memory Key 2: The epidermis, the outermost covering of the body, has five layers. The prickle-cell layer is the second deepest layer.

acanthosis thickening of the prickle-cell layer of the epidermis; may be seen in psoriasis. See Memory Key above.

accommodat/o adjust, fit

accommodation process of adjustment. Usually refers to the lens of the eye to which changes shape in order to focus a sharp image on the retina, whether the objects are near or far. For near vision, the lens becomes more rounded; for far vision, the lens becomes more flat.

acet- vinegar

Memory Key: Acet is the Roman word for vinegar. Romans noted that the hip socket was similar in shape to a vinegar cup from which they drank their wine, hence the name, *acetabulum*.

acetabular pertaining to the hip socket
acetabuloplasty surgical repair of the hip socket
acetabulum hip socket
acetylcholine a chemical released in nerve cells that permits the transmission of electrical impulses

Memory Key: In this term, **acet** means "acetic acid," **-yl** means "matter," and **choline** is a protein present in body tissues.

Achilles reflex See **reflex**.

acid- sour; sharp

acidic a compound that reacts with a base to form a salt
acidosis excess acid in the body tissues disturbing the body's acid-base balance. May be due to diabetic, pulmonary, or renal dysfunction. The opposite of acidosis is alkalosis, meaning "excess bases."

acquired immunity Production of antibodies against disease; can be passive or active. See **immun/o**.

acr/o extremities; top

acrocyanosis blue discoloration of the extremities

acrodynia pain in the extremities

acromegaly enlargement of the extremities

acrophobia fear of heights

acromi/o acromion process

acromion the spiny process projecting laterally over the shoulder joint

acromioclavicular joint the joint between the acromion process and collarbone

actin A muscle protein responsible for muscle contraction and relaxation. Found in myofilaments.

actin/o ray

actinotherapy treatment of skin disorders using rays such as ultraviolet radiation

action potential See **nerve impulse**.

ad- toward

adduct to draw toward

adduction the process of drawing a body part, such as the arm or leg, toward the midline of the body

adductor that which draws toward the midline of the body. For example the adductor muscles draw the thigh toward the midline.

adhesion bands of tissue that abnormally stick together following inflammation, usually as a result of surgery or injury. This may occur between abdominal organs, at joints, or in other areas where tissue should move about freely.

Memory Key: Adhesive tape is used to stick items together.

adnexa connecting parts of a structure. For example, uterine adnexa include the uterine tubes, ovaries, and uterine ligaments.

Memory Key 1: Adnexa is the plural. There is no singular form.

Memory Key 2: Nexa means "tie, bond, or connect" as seen in con**nec**tion and an**nexa**tion.

*a*drenal gland   endocrine gland located on top of the kidney. See **gland**. (See Appendix F, Figure 7.)
*a*drenaline   hormone secreted from the adrenal medulla. Also known as epinephrine.

Memory Key: Ad- means "toward"; **renal** refers to "kidney"; **-ine** means "chemical." Adrenaline is a chemical secreted by the adrenal medulla, which sits on top of the kidney.

*a*drenocorticotrophic hormone   substance secreted by the anterior pituitary gland to stimulate the secretion of the hormones cortisol, aldosterone, and small amounts of sex hormones from the adrenal cortex
*a*fferent   to carry toward the center. For example, an afferent artery carries blood toward the heart; an afferent neuron carries electrical impulses toward the spinal cord and brain.

Memory Key: Ad- changes to **af-** before **f**.

*a*fferent system   sensory system; see **system**

Memory Key: Ad- changes to **af-** before **f**.

aden/o gland

*a*denitis   inflammation of a gland
*a*denocarcinoma   malignant tumor of glandular tissue
*a*denohypophysis   anterior pituitary gland. See **-physis**.
*a*denoma   benign tumor of glandular tissue
*a*denopathy   glandular disease, especially enlargement of a lymph node
*a*denovirus   a large group of viruses causing upper respiratory tract infections including colds

Memory Key: The first viruses within this group were isolated in the adenoid tissue of the throat, hence the name adenovirus; **virus** means "poison."

adenoid/o adenoids

*a*denoids   pharyngeal tonsils located on the roof of the pharynx

adenoidectomy surgical excision of the adenoids

adip/o fat

***adip**ocele* hernia containing fat

***adip**ocyte* fat cells

***adip**ose* pertaining to fat

adenosine triphosphate (ATP) A chemical
found in all cells. It is especially important in muscle cells in
which energy is produced for movement when ATP is split by
enzymatic action.

adrenaline A hormone secreted by the adrenal
medulla; epinephrine.

adrenergic fibers Nerve cell fibers that release
epinephrine as a neurotransmitter.

afferent To carry toward. See Memory Key under **ad-,
afferent**.

agglutinat/o

***agglutinat**ion* the clumping of microorganisms and cells, such
as red blood cells.

agoraphobia The fear of crowded places.

alb- white

***alb**inism* lack of pigment in the skin, hair, and eyes

albino The name given to a person affected by albinism.

albumin One of several proteins found in blood plasma.

albumin/o albumin

***albumin**uria* albumin in the urine; proteinuria

-algia pain

Memory Key: Nost*algia*, meaning "homesickness," is a common English word.

arthr*algia* joint pain
ceph*algia*; cephal*algia* headache
gastr*algia* stomachache
neur*algia* nerve pain
ot*algia* earache

alimentation The giving of food or nourishment to the body. May be artificial or forced.

aliment/o nutrition

***aliment*ary tract** digestive tract

allantois Embryonic membranes that develop into the connective stalk and eventually become the umbilical cord.

allergen Any substance that can produce an allergic response.

Memory Key: **-gen** means "producing."

allergy Hypersensitive reaction to foreign proteins that do not cause a reaction in most people. Abnormal reactions include coldlike symptoms, eczema, hives, and bronchial asthma.

allo- other

***allo*graft** tissue graft between members of the same species but of different genetic backgrounds

all-or-none theory Principle applied when a motor neuron stimulates a muscle fiber; the muscle either contracts to the fullest degree possible or not at all.

alopecia Loss of hair; baldness.

alpha (α) first letter of the Greek alphabet

alpha **cells** cells in the islets of Langerhans of the pancreas that secrete the hormone glucagon. Glucagon changes glycogen to glucose.

alpha **waves** see **waves**.

alveol/o hollow; cavity

alveolitis inflammation of the pulmonary alveoli. See **alveolus** definition (1).

alveolus (1) The pulmonary alveoli through which oxygen and carbon dioxide are exchanged. (2) The cavity in which the tooth sits. Also known as the tooth socket.

ambly/o dimness

amblyopia dim or reduced vision

amni/o amnion (sac enclosing the fetus)

amniocentesis surgical puncture to remove amniotic fluid from the amnion

amniorrhexis ruptured amnion

amniotic **cavity** hollow space within the amnion filled with amniotic fluid

amniotic **fluid** fluid within the amniotic sac that protects and supports the fetus; the fetus floats in the amniotic fluid

amniotomy surgical incision of the amnion to induce labor

amnion The embryonic membrane enclosing the fetus and secreting amniotic fluid in which the embryo and later the fetus float; it protects the fetus from injury.

Memory Key: The **amnion** is also known as *the bag of waters*.

amphi- both sides

amphiarthrosis a slightly moveable joint; the surfaces of the opposing bones are connected by cartilage. For example, the symphysis pubis connects the pelvic bones anteriorly.

amyl- starch

amylase an enzyme that breaks down starch

ana- up; without; backward; apart

anabolic steroids synthetic chemical compounds that re-semble the natural male sex hormones. Used in medicine to promote the growth and repair of body tissues.

anabolism a type of metabolic process. See **-bol**.

anaphase third phase of mitosis in which each chromatid moves apart toward its respective poles to form the daughter chromosomes. Each chromatid is considered a separate chromosome.

anaphylactic shock reduced blood pressure due to an increased hypersensitivity to an allergen; may be fatal. See **shock**.

anaplasia a term applied to cancerous cells that revert to a less developed state in arrangement and structure; a loss of differentiation among cells. Also known as *dedifferentiation*.

Memory Key: Anaplasia literally means a "backward development."

anastomosis the joining of two body parts that are normally separate. For example, advanced cancer of the small intestine may necessitate its complete removal. After the small intestine is removed in its entirety, the stomach may be connected to the large intestine. This new opening or connection between the stomach and large intestine is called an *anastomosis* or a *gastrocolostomy*.

anatomy the study of the structure of the body

Memory Key 1: Anatomy literally means "to cut" (**-tomy**) "apart" (**ana-**). In order to study the body, it must be cut apart or dissected.

Memory Key 2: Note the combination of the prefix **ana-** with the suffix **-tomy**. This is different from the usual combination of a root and a suffix in creating a medical word.

andr/o male; man

androgens a group of hormones responsible for maintaining the secondary male sexual characteristics of muscle bulk, facial hair, and deep voice. Testosterone is an example.

aneurysm
A weak spot in the arterial wall will result in its widening or distention. This bulge in the arterial wall will continually stretch and widen because it is affected by the blood pressure. If not treated, the aneurysm will burst. If it occurs in the brain it will cause a stroke due to the loss of blood.

ang- distress; choke

Memory Key: Related English words are ***ang**uish* or ***anx**ious* meaning "distressing," and ***ang**er*, which originally meant "a choking pain."

***ang**ina* distressing pain
***ang**ina pectoris* chest pain that may be symptomatic of a heart attack

angi/o vessel

***angi**ectasis* dilatation of a blood vessel
***angi**itis or **ang**itis* inflammation of the blood vessel
***angi**ocardiography* a process in which an image of the heart's blood vessels is produced using x-rays following intravenous injection of a contrast medium
***angi**ography* a process in which an image of the blood vessels is produced using x-rays following intravenous injection of a contrast medium. The type of angiography is described by the preceding adjective. Examples include:
  cerebral a.: x-ray of the vascular system of the brain
  coronary a.: x-ray of the vascular system of the heart. Also known as angiocardiography.

digital subtraction a. (DSA): process of producing an x-ray image of blood vessels by subtracting background shadows that may cause poor visualization of the image. Using specialized computer software, a clearer image of the vessels is obtained as compared to the simpler angiography.

pulmonary a.: x-ray of the vessels of the lungs

angiogram record or image of a blood vessel produced by x-rays.

angioma benign tumor of blood vessels

angioplasty a clinical procedure that removes areas of constriction in a blood vessel

laser a.: a procedure in which a catheter equipped with a laser is placed into the lumen of the stenosed or obstructed coronary artery. A light beam from the laser travels to the diseased site and vaporizes the fatty material.

percutaneous transluminal a. (PTA): a surgical procedure using a balloon-tipped catheter to open a blood vessel blocked by fatty plaques. The catheter is inserted through the skin (percutaneous), across the lumen of the vessel (transluminal), to the site of obstruction. The balloon is inflated flattening the fatty plaques against the arterial wall. The blood can now flow freely through the blood vessel. The catheter is removed. A tiny support structure called a **stent** may be placed inside the artery to keep the artery open. Cells quickly grow over the stent, providing a smooth inner lining.

angiosarcoma malignant tumor of blood vessels

angiospasm sudden, involuntary contraction of the muscles associated with the blood vessels

angiostenosis narrowing of a blood vessel

angiotensin I hormone that is a precursor to angiotensin II

angiotensin II hormone that increases blood pressure

Memory Key: Tens/o means "stretched out," therefore, narrowing. Under the influence of angiotensin, the blood vessel walls narrow, increasing the blood pressure.

anion An ion carrying a negative electrical charge.

anis/o unequal size; variation in size

anisocoria inequality in the size of the pupils

anisocytosis increased variation in the size of cells, particularly red blood cells

ankle jerk See **reflex, Achilles**.

ankyl/o fusion of parts; bent; crooked; stiff

ankyloglossia tongue tied

ankylosing spondylitis a form of arthritis affecting the vertebrae, which may lead to fusion of the spinal joints

ankylosis fusion and immobility of a joint due to surgery, disease, or injury

annul/o ring

annulus fibrosus a fibrous ring surrounding the nucleus pulposus of the intervertebral disc

Memory Key: Relate **annulus,** "a circular ring," to **annual** meaning "a circular journey."

an/o anus

Memory Key: **An/o** is most likely related to **annul/o** meaning "a ring" because the anus is a circular structure.

anal sphincter see sphincter

anoperineal pertaining to the anus and perineum

Memory Key: Do not confuse *perineum* with *peritoneum*. The perineum is an area around the genitals; the peritoneum is a membrane in the abdominal cavity.

anorectal pertaining to the anus and rectum

anoscopy process of visually examining the anus with a scope

anus lower part of the rectum. (See Appendix F, Figure 6.)

Memory Key: **-us** is a noun ending.

ante- before

ante **cibum (a.c.)** before meals. Commonly used in prescriptions to tell patients when to take their medication.

anteflexion forward bending of a body part. Compare with **retroflexion**.

antenatal before birth with reference to the fetus; prenatal

antepartum; ante **partum** before birth with reference to the mother.

anteversion forward tilting of a body part. Compare with **retroversion**.

anter/o front

anterior pertaining to the front of a body part

anterior **cavity** space in front of the lens of the eye filled with aqueous humor

anterior **chamber** portion of the eye's anterior cavity between the iris and lens

anterior **column** anterior portion of the white matter on either side of the spinal cord. Also known as *ventral column*.

anterior **horn** anterior projection of gray matter of the spinal cord. Also known as *ventral horn*.

anterior **root** one of two roots by which a spinal nerve is attached to the spinal cord. Emerging from the union between the anterior and posterior root is the spinal nerve. Also known as *ventral root*.

anterior **pituitary gland** see **gland, pituitary**.

anteroposterior from the front to the back. In radiology, the anteroposterior (AP) position refers to x-rays projected through the body structure from the front to the back.

anthracosis A condition in which inhaled coal dust from coal mining lines the walls of the alveoli making the exchange of oxygen and carbon dioxide difficult; also known as black lung disease.

anti- against

antacids agents that neutralize hydrochloric acid

antibiotics drugs used to prevent the growth or life of a disease-causing microorganism. Example: penicillin.

antianginal drug used to relieve chest pain or angina

antiarrhythmics drugs used to suppress various types of abnormal cardiac rhythms

antibody a protein produced by the body in response to foreign substances (antigens) such as bacteria, viruses, and other toxins. When the antibody specifically combines with the antigen that stimulated its production (antigen-antibody reaction), the harmful effects of the invading microorganism are neutralized.

anticholinergic (1) Inhibition of the parasympathetic nervous system. (2) Drugs used to block the action of the parasympathetic nervous system. Actions include a decrease of all secretions, reduced gastrointestinal and genitourinary motility, and dilatation of pupils.

Memory Key: **-cholin** refers to acetylcholine, a neurotransmitter released at parasympathetic nerve endings.

anticoagulants drugs used to prevent the formation of clots

anticonvulsants drugs used to prevent convulsions (seizures)

antidiuretic hormone hormone produced by the hypothalamus and secreted by the posterior pituitary to inhibit urine excretion. Also known as vasopressin.

Memory Key: **Dia** means "through"; **ure/o** means "urine."

antidote a chemical that works against a poison. **Dote** means "to give."

antiemetics drugs used to relieve vomiting. For example Phenergan.

antiflatulents drugs that reduce gastric bloating

antigen foreign substances such as viruses, bacteria or other toxins that stimulate the production of antibodies

Memory Key: **Antigen** is short for **antibody generator**.

antigen-antibody reaction following the production of the antibody by the antigen, the antibody combines specifically with the antigen, rendering the antigen harmless

antiglobulin an antibody that reacts against gamma globulins (Ig). In an antiglobulin test, certain conditions are diagnosed by identifying whether the erythrocytes are coated with antibodies; useful in diagnosing diseases including hemolytic anemia, renal disorders, and hemolytic disease of the newborn.

antihistamines drugs that work against the action of histamine and reduce uncomfortable symptoms of redness, swelling, heat, and pain caused by the release of histamine in response to antigens entering the body. See **histamine**.

antihypertensives drugs used to alleviate high blood pressure

anti-inflammatory drugs drugs used to treat inflammatory conditions characterized by redness, swelling, heat, and pain.

antineoplastics drugs that work against the growth or spread of malignant cells

antinuclear antibodies (ANA) antibodies the body produces against its own nuclear material. Their presence indicates autoimmune diseases such as systemic lupus erythematosus and rheumatoid arthritis.

antipruritics drugs that relieve itching. Examples include Calamine and benzocaine.

antipsychotics drugs used to relieve symptoms of psychoses, such as hallucinations

antipyretics drugs used to reduce fevers. Examples include aspirin and Tylenol.

antiseptic an agent that impedes the growth of a disease-producing microorganism

antispasmodics drugs that relieve violent involuntary muscle spasms

antitoxin poisonous substance secreted by living bacterial cells

antitussives drugs that relieve coughing. Example is Benylin.

anus The opening of the rectum at the end of the digestive tract. (See Appendix F, Figure 6.)

aort/o aorta

aorta the largest artery in the body from which smaller arteries branch to the internal organs; carries oxygenated blood to body tissues. (See Appendix F, Figure 1.)

Memory Key: Aor is a word element that means "to rise up." The aorta is the largest artery in the body and rises up from the heart.

aortic aneurysm a bulging of the walls of the aorta

Memory Key: Note the use of the adjectival ending **-ic**.

aortic semilunar valve see **valve**

aortitis inflammation of the aorta

aortoiliac pertaining to the aorta and iliac artery

aortography process of producing x-ray images of the aorta

aortorrhaphy to stitch or suture the aorta

aortostenosis narrowing of the aorta

apex Point of an angle, cone, or pyramid.

apex of heart: pointed inferior portion of the heart

apex of lung: pointed superior portion of the lung

apo- away from; derived from

apocrine gland glands that lose some of their cellular structure when secreting their product. **-crine** means "to secrete." See **gland.**

aponeurosis broad, flat tendinous attachment connecting muscle to bone. An example is the galea **apo**neurotica on the top of the head connecting the skull muscles.

Memory Key: Do not take neurosis to mean neuron or a psychological condition. In this case, **neurosis** refers to a tendon. Early anatomists applied the term neuron to any rounded, white structure; both nerves and tendons fit into this category. It was sometime later that the root **neur/o** was applied to nerves only.

appendicular skeleton
Bones attached to the trunk as appendages; included are the bones of the arms and legs.

appendix
Structure of the digestive system that hangs onto the cecum; vermiform appendix. (See Appendix F, Figure 6.)

Memory Key: The word *appendix* can be divided into **ap-** meaning "to" or "on" and **-pendix** meaning "hanging part." The appendix is a structure that hangs onto the cecum.

append/o appendix
***append*ectomy** surgical excision of the appendix
***append*icitis** inflammation of the appendix

aque/o water
***aque*ous humor** a watery fluid produced in the eye that circulates through the anterior and posterior chambers and drains into the venous system through the canal of Schlemm. It functions to refract (bend) light rays.

arachn/o spider
***arachn*oid membrane** the middle layer of the meninges resembling a spider web. See **mening/o, meninges**.
***arachn*oid villi** fingerlike projections of the arachnoid membrane

arteri/o artery
***arteri*al** pertaining to an artery
***arteri*ogram** a record or image of the artery produced by x-rays
***arteri*ography** process of producing an x-ray image of an artery following injection of a contrast medium
***arteri*ole** small artery
***arteri*opathy** any disease of the artery
***arteri*orrhaphy** suture of the artery

Memory Key: Remember, **-rrhaphy** has two Rs.

arteriorrhexis rupture of the artery

Memory Key: Remember, **-rrhexis** has two Rs.

arteriosclerosis hardening of the artery. See Memory Key under **arteriostenosis**.

arteriostenosis narrowing of the artery

Memory Key: Differentiate **-stenosis** from **-sclerosis** by remembering that a **steno**grapher is someone who writes in shorthand; therefore narrowing or shortening the English language.

arteritis inflammation of the artery

artery
A blood vessel that carries blood away from the heart. All arteries except the pulmonary artery carry oxygenated blood.

arthr/o joint

arthralgia joint pain; arthrodynia

arthritis inflammation of a joint. Two common types of arthritides are:

osteoarthritis: noninflammatory joint disease characterized by the wearing away of articular cartilage causing friction between bones that results in pain and stiffness; degenerative arthritis

rheumatoid a.: inflammation of connective tissue, which may affect joints throughout the entire body; thought to be an autoimmune disease that can progress to fusion and immobility of the joint

arthrocentesis surgical puncture of a joint to remove fluid

arthrodesis surgical procedure that locks the joint in one position, thereby reducing pain; surgical fusion of a joint.

arthrodynia joint pain, arthralgia

arthrogram record of a joint made by x-rays following injection of a contrast medium

arthropathy any disease of a joint

arthroplasty surgical repair of a joint; usually refers to the total or partial replacement of the knee or hip joints with a prosthetic (artificial) device

arthroscope instrument used to view inside a joint cavity

arthroscopy process of visually examining the joint cavity using an arthroscope. In arthroscopic surgery, a video camera takes images of a joint cavity and displays these images on a TV monitor. With this technique, the joint can be worked on under local anesthetic with good visualization of the entire joint. Recovery time is minimal and hospital stay reduced.

arthrosis abnormal condition of a joint

arthrotomy incision into a joint

articul/o joint

articular cartilage smooth material found at joint surfaces

asbestosis
A form of lung disease caused by inhaling asbestos-dust particles that consequently line the walls of the pulmonary alveoli, making the exchange of oxygen and carbon dioxide difficult.

ascites
The abnormal accumulation of excess fluid in the peritoneal cavity, most commonly caused by cirrhosis of the liver due to alcoholism but also from heart failure and kidney disease.

-ase enzyme

amylase enzyme that breaks down starch

lactase enzyme that converts glucose to galactose

lipase enzyme that changes fats into fatty acids and glycerol

maltase enzyme that converts maltose to glucose

peptidase digestive enzyme secreted by the small intestine that converts peptides to amino acids

phenylalanine hydroxylase enzyme necessary to change phenylalanine to tyrosine; lack of this enzyme results in increased phenylalanine in the blood that eventually spills over into the urine. See **phenylketonuria**.

phosphodiesterase enzyme that degrades cyclic adenosine monophosphate (cAMP)

protease enzyme that breaks down protein

sucrase enzyme secreted by the small intestine to break sucrose into glucose and fructose

aspiration (1) To withdraw fluid, air, or tissue from a cavity. For example, fluid may be **aspirated** from the peritoneal cavity in ascites; air may be **aspirated** from the pleural cavity; bone marrow may be **aspirated** from the medullary cavity, and fluid may be **aspirated** from a joint cavity. In all these cases, a needle is placed into the cavity and the specific substance aspirated or withdrawn. (2) To inhale as in **aspiration pneumonia,** in which the patient has aspirated or inhaled vomitus into the lung.

Memory Key: Aspirate comes from the Latin **-ad** meaning "toward" and **spir/o** meaning "to breathe," hence to breathe toward. In aspiration pneumonia, the patient inhales the vomitus into the lungs.

asthma Reversible bronchospasm that obstructs the small airways and produces shortness of breath.

status *asthmaticus* a prolonged bronchospasm in which the bronchus fails to relax following treatment with bronchodilators; may be fatal

astigmatism Error of refraction due to the defective curvature of the cornea or lens of the eye, preventing light rays from focussing on the same point on the retina, thus causing impaired vision.

atel/o incomplete

atelectasis (1) Inability of the alveoli to completely inflate due to bronchial obstruction. (2) Collapsed lung due to external pressure on the lung or, in newborns, due to a reduction in surfactant.

ather/o fatty plaque

atheroma fatty mass or debris that accumulates on arterial walls, gradually narrowing the arterial lumen

atherosclerosis accumulation of fatty debris (**atheroma**) on the inner arterial wall; a type of arteriosclerosis

atlas
The first cervical vertebra (C1) that holds the head on top of the spinal column. (See Appendix F, Figure 21.)

Memory Key: Atlas was a Greek god whose duty was to hold the world on his shoulders. The atlas (C1) holds up the skull.

atri/o atrium

***atrial* fibrillation** abnormal heart beat affecting the atrium, characterized by very fast, irregular, uncoordinated heart beats of approximately 300 to 400 beats per minute

***atrio*ventricular (AV) bundle** see **conduction system**

***atrio*ventricular node (AV) node** see **conduction system**

***atrio*ventricular (AV) valve** (See Appendix F, Figure 4.)

inter*atri*al septum wall separating the right and left atria

Memory Key: Septum means "wall" or "fence"

atrium upper right and left chambers of the heart. Plural is atria. (See Appendix F, Figure 4.)

Memory Key: An **atrium** is an entrance hall where guests are received. The **atria** of the heart are like entrance halls in that they are the first to receive blood before the blood flows to the ventricles.

audi/o hearing

***audi*ogram** record of a patient's hearing ability

***audi*ometer** instrument used to measure hearing

***audi*ometry** process of measuring a patient's hearing ability

audit/o hearing

***audit*ory** pertaining to hearing

***audit*ory tube** eustachian tube

auris dexter (AD) The right ear. *Auris* (ear); *dexter* (right).

auris sinistra (AS) The left ear. *Auris* (ear); *sinistra* (left).

aur/o ear

aural pertaining to the ear

Memory Key: Do not confuse **aural** with *oral*, meaning pertaining to the mouth.

auricle the external ear; the pinna

auscult/o listen

auscultation the process of listening to sounds within the body. A stethoscope is used to listen to breath sounds, heart sounds, and bowel sounds. Auscultation is one of four techniques used during the physical examination as an aid to diagnosis. The other techniques include inspection, palpation (feeling), and percussion (tapping). Together with auscultation, the entire process can be abbreviated IPPA.

auto- self

autograft transplant of tissue from one part of the patient's body to another

autoimmune disease an immune response to one's own body tissue; destruction of one's own cells by the immune system. Rheumatoid arthritis and systemic lupus erythematosus are examples of autoimmune diseases.

autopsy internal and external examination of the body following death to determine its cause. Also known as *postmortem examination* or *necropsy*.

axill/o armpit; axilla

axillary pertaining to the armpit

axillary node lymph node located under the armpit. See **lymph nodes**.

axis The second cervical vertebra (C2) on which the head rotates. (See Appendix F, Figure 21.)

Memory Key: Extending from the body of C2 is a toothlike projection known as the *dens* or *odontoid process*. This process or projection allows the head to rotate on its axis.

axon The part of a neuron (nerve cell) that transmits electrical impulses away from the cell body; an elongated nerve fiber. (See Appendix F, Figure 13.)

axon terminal See **synaptic knob**.

azotemia Uremia. See **ur/o, uremia**.

B

Babinski's reflex See **reflex**.

backbone See **spin/o, spinal column**.

bacteri/o bacteria

bacteremia bacteria in the blood
bacterial pertaining to bacteria
bactericidal agent that kills bacteria
bacteriology study of bacteria
bacteriuria bacteria in the urine

balan/o glans penis

balanitis inflammation of the glans penis
balanorrhea discharge or flow from the glans penis

barium studies
X-ray examination of the gastrointestinal tract (GIT). Barium, a chalky-tasting, thick liquid, is used as a contrast medium to highlight the organs of the GIT when seen on x-rays. Types include:

barium enema: x-ray and fluoroscopic examination of the lower gastrointestinal tract

barium swallow: x-ray and fluoroscopic examination of the pharynx and esophagus

small bowel follow through: x-ray and fluoroscopic examination of the small bowel. Pictures are taken at specific time intervals following the barium as it progresses through the small intestine.

small bowel series: x-ray and fluoroscopic examination of the duodenum, ileum, and jejunum

upper gastrointestinal series: x-ray and fluoroscopic examination of the pharynx, esophagus, stomach, and proximal duodenum

bar/o weight; pressure; heavy

baroreceptor nerve receptor sensitive to changes in blood pressure. Baroreceptors located in blood vessel walls will respond to changes in blood pressure by constricting or dilating the vessel walls.

Memory Key: Think of a *barometer*, an instrument used to indicate the weight of the atmosphere.

barotitis media inflammation of the middle ear caused by changes in atmospheric pressure that can occur in a descending airplane or in deep-sea diving

Bartholin's glands
Two small glands located on either side of the vaginal orifice. These glands secrete a fluid that lubricates the vagina, preparing it for intercourse.

bartholinitis inflammation of Bartholin's glands

Memory Key: Note that **Bartholin's gland** is capitalized but **bartholinitis** is not. This is because Bartholin is an eponym, a name for a disease, structure, place, or surgical procedure named after a particular person; bartholinitis is an adaptation of the person's name and is therefore not capitalized.

***Bartholin's* abscess** accumulation of pus in a Bartholin's gland due to an infection with pyogenic bacteria such as streptococci or staphylococci

***Bartholin's* cyst** a closed sac within a Bartholin's gland containing a fluid, semifluid, or solid material

bas/o base; bottom level; nonacidic

***basal* cell carcinoma** malignant tumor of the basal (deepest) cell layer of the epidermis; metastasis is rare

***basal* ganglia** islands of gray matter embedded in the white matter deep in the cerebrum. Basal ganglia are important in controlling motor functions. Also known as *basal nuclei.*

***basal* metabolic rate (BMR)** the rate at which energy is used for basic metabolic processes of the body only. Base conditions are set up for testing. For example, the test is given after a good sleep, 12 to 14 hours after eating, no previous exercise or excitement, and at a normal body temperature. Measured in kilocalories per hour.

***basal* nuclei** see **bas/o, basal ganglia**

***baso*phil** type of white blood cell. See **-phil**.

basement membrane A membrane underlying a
layer of epithelial cells, serving as support and attachment.

B-cell A type of white blood cell. See **B-lymphocyte.**

bedsore An open sore caused by lying in one position
for too long. Also known as **decubitis ulcer**. See **ulcer**.

Bell's palsy Paralysis of one side of the face involving
the facial nerve (7th cranial nerve).

Bence-Jones protein A protein found in the urine
of patients with multiple myeloma.

benign Noncancerous; not harmful. When cells are said to be **benign** they are differentiated, encapsulated, and do not metastasize (spread). Compare with **malignant**.

benign prostatic hypertrophy (BPH) benign enlargement of the prostate usually occurring in men over 50 years of age. As the prostate enlarges, it squeezes the urethra, obstructing the passage of urine.

beta (β) second letter in the Greek alphabet

beta blockers one of several drugs used to vasodilate blood vessels and to reduce the heart rate by blocking certain receptors in the autonomic nervous system

beta cells cells that produce the hormone insulin, which changes glucose to glycogen. These cells are located in the islets of Langerhans of the pancreas.

beta waves see **wave**

bi- two

biceps having two heads or divisions

biceps brachii muscle of the upper arm. (See Appendix F, Figure 9.) See **-ceps**.

bicuspid having two points or projections

bicuspid tooth a bicuspid tooth has two projections. Also known as *premolars*.

bicuspid valve heart valve between the left atrium and ventricle; also known as the mitral or atrioventricular valve. (See Appendix F, Figure 4.).

bifurcation division of a structure into two parts. For example, the trachea bifurcates into the right and left bronchi.

bilateral pertaining to two sides. For example, the lungs are bilateral.

bipolar neuron a nerve cell that has two processes (axons and dendrites) extending from each end of the cell body. (See Appendix F, Figure 13)

bisection cutting into two parts

bile A substance produced in the liver and stored in the gallbladder for the purpose of breaking down fats in the duodenum. When bile is needed to break down fats, it must travel from the gallbladder to the duodenum by a system of ducts called the *biliary tract.*

bil/i   bile; gall

biliary atresia closure of one or more of the biliary ducts

Memory Key: -tresia means "opening"; **a-** means "no" or "not."

biliary calculi gallstones; stones located in the gallbladder or anywhere along the biliary tract

biliary tract liver, gallbladder, hepatic ducts, cystic ducts, common bile ducts, and other structures that participate in the delivery of bile from the liver to the duodenum

bilirubin an orange-yellow bile pigment derived from the breakdown of hemoglobin in old red blood cells. Bilirubin passes in the bile into the duodenum where it is excreted in the feces.

bi/o   life

biology the study of life and living organisms

biopsy microscopic examination of living tissue for abnormalities. Types include:

conization b.: procedure in which a cone-shaped piece of tissue is removed for examination; often performed on the cervix uteri

excisional b.: removal of the entire suspected lesion for microscopic examination

incisional b.: removal of a small segment of the suspected lesion for microscopic examination

needle b.: a procedure in which deep tissue can be obtained for examination by piercing the skin with a needle, withdrawing the tissue, and bringing it to the surface in its lumen

punch b.: a procedure in which a circular piece of tissue is removed for examination; usually performed on the cervix uteri

-blast immature stage; growing thing

erythro*blast* immature red blood cell
leuko*blast* immature white blood cell
megalo*blast* immature abnormal red blood cell with a large-
  sized nucleus. May be found in cases of pernicious anemia.

blast/o shoot; bud

***blast*ocele** normal, fluid-filled cavity within the blastocyst (part
  of the developing embryo). Also spelled *blastocoele*. See
  blastocyst.
***blast*ocyst** one of the stages in the developing embryo
  formed by continuous cell division of the fertilized ovum. It
  consists of cells that develop into embryonic membranes,
  other cells that develop into a new individual, and a fluid-
  filled cavity called a **blastocele**. It is the **blastocyst** that
  implants itself onto the uterine wall for further development
  into a fetus.

bleb See **bulla**.

blephar/o eyelid

***blephar*ochalasis** drooping of the eyelid. **-chalasis** means
  "relaxation."
***blephar*opexy** surgical fixation of the eyelid
***blephar*optosis** drooping of the eyelid
***blephar*ospasm** sudden involuntary muscle contraction of
  the eyelid

blood Fluid that circulates through the heart and blood
vessels to nourish organs and remove waste products; consists
of plasma and blood cells.

blood-brain barrier A protective mechanism that
prevents toxic substances from entering the brain, while at the
same time allowing needed substances such as glucose and
oxygen to enter.

blood pressure The force exerted by blood on the
blood vessel wall. Includes **diastolic pressure**, which is the

pressure against the arterial walls when the ventricles are relaxing and **systolic pressure**, which is pressure on the arterial walls when the ventricles contract.

B-lymphocyte Cells that are produced in the bone marrow and that travel to the lymph nodes and other lymphoid tissue to become part of the body's immune system. B-lymphocytes produce antibodies to combat antigens. The antibodies produced are called *immunoglobulins* (Ig), such as IgM, IgD, IgA, IgE, IgG. Also known as *B-cells*.

-bol throw

ana*bol*ism metabolic process in which complex substances are built up from less complex ones. An example is the combining of amino acids to form protein.

cata*bol*ism metabolic process in which complex substances are broken into simpler substances. An example is the breaking down of complex proteins into simpler amino acids.

em*bol*us a blood clot or foreign clump of material that has detached from the blood vessel wall and moves through the blood stream becoming stuck in the vessel and obstructing blood flow

Memory Key: Embolus comes from Greek **embolos** meaning "plug." An embolos was used as a cork in a liquor bottle.

meta*bol*ism chemical and physical changes that occur in the body including catabolism and anabolism

bolus (1) A rounded, softened mass of chewed food ready to be swallowed. (2) A concentrated pharmaceutical preparation, such as a contrast medium, given intravenously for diagnostic purposes.

bone scan A diagnostic procedure utilizing a radioactive substance and a gamma camera. See **scan**.

bony labyrinth The bony structure of the inner ear. See **labyrinth**.

bowel The intestines, including small and large intestines. Also known as the *gut*.

Memory Key: The word **bowel** is Latin meaning "sausage."

bow-legged See **genu, genu varum**.

Bowman's capsule Structure found in the nephron. See **glomerular capsule**.

brachi/o arm
brachial plexus a network of nerves in the arm. See **plexus**.
brachiocephalic pertaining to the arm and head

brady- slow
bradycardia abnormally slow heart beat
bradykinesia slow movement
bradyphrasia slow speech
bradypnea slow breathing

brain scan A diagnostic procedure utilizing a radioactive substance and a gamma camera. See **scan**.

Braxton-Hicks contraction See **contraction**.

breech presentation In obstetrics, presentation refers to the part of the fetus that is felt through the cervix at time of delivery. **Breech presentation** refers to the buttocks presenting themselves through the cervix.

bronchi/o bronchus
bronchial pertaining to the bronchus
bronchiectasis dilatation of the bronchus
bronchiole smaller subdivisions of the bronchus

bronchitis inflammation of the bronchus

bronchodilator drugs that relax the muscles of the bronchus to alleviate bronchospasm and to increase air flow into the lungs. Used as a symptomatic treatment in such conditions as asthma.

bronchogenic carcinoma malignant tumor of the lung originating from the bronchus

bronchopneumonia inflammation of the lungs and terminal bronchioles

bronchoscopy process of visually examining the bronchus with the aid of a bronchoscope

bronchospasm sudden, violent muscular contraction of the bronchus

bronchus Respiratory passage carrying air from the trachea to the lungs.

bucc/o cheek

buccal mucosa pertaining to the mucous membrane of the cheek. **Mucosa** is another term for *mucous membrane*.

buccal cavity mouth or oral cavity

bulbourethral gland A gland of the male reproductive system. See **gland**. (See Appendix F, Figure 17.)

bulimia An eating disorder characterized by patterns of binge eating followed by self-induced vomiting.

bulla A large blister (vesicle), greater than 1 cm in diameter, containing serous (watery) or seropurulent (watery and pus-filled) fluid. Also called a *bleb*. Appears as an abnormal condition of the lung or epidermis.

bundle branches A portion of the conduction system branching from the bundle of His. See **conduction system**. (See Appendix F, Figure 3.)

bunion An inward, bony projection of the first metatarsal accompanied by the displacement of the great toe away from the midline.

burs/o bursa

Memory Key: Bursa is a Greek term meaning "leather pouch." A *bursar* is a college treasurer in the sense of keeping the money in a leather pouch.

bursa sac filled with synovial fluid located around joints

Memory Key: -a is a noun ending.

bursectomy excision of the bursa
bursitis inflammation of the bursa

CABG Coronary artery bypass graft. See under **coron/o**.

calcane/o heel
***calcane*al** pertaining to the heel
***calcane*us** heel bone. One of seven bones making up the ankle. Also known as *os calcis*. See **tarsal bones**.

Memory Key: Note the noun ending **-us**. Be careful not to spell the word as *calcane**ous***. There is no such term.

calc/o calcium; limestone
***calc*ium** see **mineral**

calcitonin a hormone secreted by the parafollicular cells of the thyroid gland to regulate the level of blood calcium

calculus abnormal stone or stones formed in the body organs from mineral salts. The organs most often affected are the kidneys, ureters, and gallbladder. Plural is *calculi.*

Memory Key: Calculus literally means "a small limestone pebble." Because pebbles were used at one time for counting, we now have the words *calculate* and *calculus,* a branch of mathematics.

calic/o, cali/o, calyc/o, caly/o calix; calyx

caliceal pertaining to the renal calix. Also spelled calyceal.

caliectasis dilatation of the renal calix. Also spelled calyectasis.

calix, calyx A cup-shaped organ or cavity. Plural is *calices* or *calyces.* The **renal calices** are subdivisions of the renal pelvis through which urine passes on its way to the bladder. Includes the **major** and **minor calices**.

callus A localized thickening and hardening of the top layer of the epidermis due to friction and pressure.

cAMP Cyclic adenosine monophosphate. A substance that regulates the activity of important enzymes.

canal of Schlemm The space between the sclera and cornea of the eye, which drains aqueous humor from the anterior cavity. (See Appendix F, Figure 15.)

cancellous bone Bony tissue that has a latticework appearance. Also known as *spongy bone.*

candid/o glowing white

Candida albicans the microorganism that most frequently causes candidiasis; a fungus

candidiasis a fungal infection caused by the genus *Candida*. Manifests itself as white patches on the mucous membrane of the mouth and vagina; yeast infection. Also known as *moniliasis*.

capillary Tiny blood vessels that link arterioles with venules. They function to exchange nutrients and waste products between the blood and tissue fluid.

capitate One of eight carpal bones. See **carpal bones** under **carp/o**.

carbon 13 (^{13}C) See **radioisotope**.

carbuncle An inflammation of skin and subcutaneous tissue characterized by a cluster of pyogenic (pus producing) boils.

Memory Key: carbuncle is Latin for "little coal" or "charcoal."

carcin/o cancer

carcinogenic agent that produces cancer

Memory Key: The word **cancer** comes from Latin meaning "crab." A cancer that has metastasized (spread) is like the claws of a crab that reach out.

carcinoma malignant tumor of epithelial cells
carcinoma in situ a premalignant neoplasm that has not invaded the basement membrane but shows cytologic characteristics of cancer; cancer cells that have not invaded neighboring tissues.

cardi/o heart

cardiac arrest sudden stoppage of the heart from pumping out blood; results in the stoppage of circulation
cardiac cycle series of consecutive movements in one heart beat in which simultaneous contraction of the atria is followed by simultaneous contraction of the ventricles
cardiac muscle heart muscle. See **muscle**.

cardiac scan a diagnostic procedure utilizing a radioactive substance and a gamma camera. See **scan**.

cardiac sphincter circular muscle at the distal end of the esophagus. See **sphincter**.

cardiogenic shock sudden reduction in blood pressure due to heart failure. See **shock**.

cardiograph instument used to record the heartbeat

cardiologist a specialist in the study of heart disease

cardiology the study of the heart

cardiomegaly abnormal enlargement of the heart

cardiomyopathy any disease of the heart muscle or myocardium

cardioplegia paralysis of the heart. The temporary and deliberate interruption of the heart's impulses, usually for the purposes of performing surgery on the heart.

cardiopulmonary bypass use of a mechanical device to take over the function of the heart and lungs during heart surgery. One segment of the device oxygenates the blood, the other segment pumps the blood through the body.

cardiovascular system See **system**.

cardiopulmonary resuscitation (CPR) a procedure involving artificial respiration and the external massage of the heart to restore cardiac function following cardiac arrest

cardiorrhexis ruptured heart

cardioversion the use of an electrical shock to restore the heart to its normal rhythm. Also known as *defibrillation*.

carditis inflammation of the heart

caries The decay and degeneration of bone. For example **dental caries** means "tooth decay."

carina A half-moon projection on the trachea located where the trachea bifurcates (divides) into the two main bronchi.

Memory Key: Carina is Latin for "keel of a boat" and has come to mean a projection or ridge.

carotene A yellow pigment found in body tissue; a red-orange hydrocarbon found in beets and carrots.

Memory Key: Do not confuse *carotene* with keratin, which is a protein found in the epidermis.

carp/o wrist

***carp*us** the wrist

Memory Key: Note the noun ending **-us**.

***carp*al bones** bones of the wrist, which include hamate, pisiform, triquetral, lunate, trapezium, trapezoid, capitate, and scaphoid. (See Appendix F, Figure 19.)

Memory Key: Note the adjectival ending, **-al**, in carp**al** and compare it to the noun ending, **-us**, in carp**us**.

meta*carp*al pertaining to bones of the hand

Memory Key: The prefix **meta** means "beyond." The bones of the hand are *beyond* the wrist.

***carp*al tunnel syndrome (CTS)** compression of the median nerve as it passes down the forearm and through the carpal tunnel. Compression, often due to overuse of a keyboard; results in pain and abnormal sensations.

***carp*optosis** wrist drop. A condition in which the hand is bent at the wrist and is unable to be extended. Wrist drop is caused by muscle or nerve damage to the area.

cartilage   A type of connective tissue that is white, tough, and avascular.

Memory Key: Cartilage comes from Latin meaning "gristle." The gristle you see on the top of a chicken drumstick is cartilage.

catabolism   A type of metabolic process. See **-bol**.

catecholamines   The adrenal medulla produces the hormones adrenaline (epinephrine) and noradrenaline (norepinephrine). These hormones are collectively called *catecholamines*.

catheterization The use of a catheter (flexible tube) for insertion into a body cavity for the instillation or withdrawal of fluid. Types include:

cardiac c.: insertion of a catheter into a vein, sliding it upward into the heart to obtain diagnostic information, such as cardiac output; levels of oxygen and carbon dioxide; pressures inside the atria and ventricles; and valvular, arterial, and myocardial disease. X-ray images are also taken to show heart structure following injection of contrast medium into the heart chambers.

urinary c.: the placement of the catheter into the bladder via the urethra to withdraw urine

cation An ion with a positive charge of electricity.

CAT scan Computed axial tomography. See **tom/o, tomography**.

caud/o tail

cauda equina literally means "a horse's tail"; a bundle of spinal nerves that emerge from the first lumbar vertebrae resembling a horse's tail

caudal a directional term meaning *toward the tail; inferior*

cavity a hollow space within the body. Can be normal as in the **abdominal** or **cranial cavities**; or it can be abnormal as a **cyst**.

cec/o cecum

cecal pertaining to the cecum

Memory Key: Note the adjectival ending **-al**.

cecopexy surgical fixation of the cecum

cecum first segment of the large intestine situated in the right lower quadrant. (See Appendix F, Figure 6.)

Memory Key: Note the noun ending **-um**.

-cele hernia (protrusion or displacement of an organ through a structure that normally contains it); swelling; cavity

blastocele normal fluid-filled cavity within a blastocyst; blastocoele

cystocele hernia of the bladder; protrusion or displacement of the bladder onto the vaginal wall

hematocele accumulation of blood around the testicles

hydrocele accumulation of fluid around the testicles.

meningomyelocele displacement of the meninges and spinal cord through a defect in the vertebra

rectocele protrusion or displacement of the rectum onto the vaginal wall

cell The smallest unit of life; groups of cells unite to become body tissues. Cells are differentiated, that is, each group of cells is capable of performing its own function.

cell body The central part of a cell containing the nucleus.

cell-mediated immunity See **immunity**.

cell membrane The structure that encloses the cell, giving the cell shape. Some membranes are elongated, others are spherical. Also known as *plasma membrane*.

cell respiration The name for energy production in the cell involving oxygen, carbon dioxide, glucose, ATP, water, and heat.

-centesis surgical puncture to remove fluid

abdominocentesis surgical puncture of the peritoneal cavity to remove fluid. Also known as *paracentesis*.

amniocentesis surgical puncture to remove amniotic fluid from the amnion

Memory Key: The **amnion** is the protective sac that surrounds the fetus.

arthrocentesis surgical puncture of a joint to remove fluid
thoracocentesis surgical puncture to remove fluid from the
    pleural cavity. Also known as *pleuracentesis* and *thoracentesis*.

central nervous system
The portion of the nervous system that includes the brain and spinal cord.

centrioles
Two cylindrical organelles built from microtubules and located in the centrosome. They function to organize the formation of the spindle in cell division.

centrosome
The center of the cell, which contains the centrioles.

cephal/o head
*ceph*al**algia;** *ceph*al**gia** headache
*ceph*alo**dymia** headache
*ceph*alo**pelvic disproportion** a complication of pregnancy
    in which the pelvic outlet is smaller than the size of the fetal
    head, making a vaginal delivery difficult

-ceps head
biceps having two heads or divisions
biceps **brachii** muscle of the anterior upper arm having two
    heads or divisions that attach onto the scapula. Often re-
    ferred to simply as *biceps*. (See Appendix F, Figure 9.)

Memory Key: Biceps is singular despite the "s" on the end.
There is no such word as *bicep*. This also applies to **quadriceps** and **triceps** below.

quadriceps having four heads or subdivisions
quadriceps **femoris** anterior muscle of the upper leg com-
    posed of four smaller muscles (rectus femoris, vastus lateralis,
    vastus medialis, and vastus intermedius), which work together
    to extend the leg. Often referred to simply as *quadriceps*. See
    Memory Key under **biceps branchi**.
triceps having three heads or subdivisions

triceps brachii the muscle belly of the triceps, located on the posterior upper arm, splits into three divisions or heads. Often referred to simply as *triceps*. See Memory Key under **biceps branchi**. (See Appendix F, Figure 10.)

cerebell/o cerebellum

cerebellar pertaining to the cerebellum
cerebellitis inflammation of the cerebellum
cerebellum literally means "little brain" and as such is that part of the brain that is tucked under the much larger cerebrum. (See Appendix F, Figure 11.)

cerebr/o cerebrum

cerebral angiography see **angiography**
cerebral aqueduct a canal in the midbrain connecting the third and fourth ventricles and containing cerebrospinal fluid
cerebral cortex thin layer of gray matter covering the outside of the cerebrum
cerebrovascular accident (CVA) interruption of the blood supply to the brain due to hemorrhage, ruptured aneurysm, or obstruction in the blood vessel from a thrombus or embolus. Also known as a *stroke*.
cerebral ventricles four cavities within the cerebrum containing cerebrospinal fluid
cerebrospinal fluid (CSF) watery fluid continually circulating through the ventricles of the brain, the central canal of the spinal cord, and in the subarachnoid space. CSF protects the brain and spinal cord.
cerebrum that largest and main portion of the brain. (See Appendix F, Figure 11.)

cerumen A waxy substance secreted by the external ear.

cerumin/o wax

ceruminous pertaining to cerumen
Memory Key: Note the difference in spelling between the noun cerumen with an **e** and the adjective ceruminous with an **i**.

cervic/o neck of the body; narrow or necklike portion of a structure such as the uterus

cervical plexus network of nerves in the neck. See **plexus**.

cervical vertebrae spinal bones of the neck. (See Appendix F, Figure 21.) See **vertebra**.

cervicitis inflammation of the neck of the uterus

cervix   The neck of the uterus; cervix uteri.

cheil/o lip

cheiloplasty surgical reconstruction of the lips due to congenital malformation, injury, or disease

cheilorrhaphy suturing of the lips

cheilosis abnormal condition of the lips characterized by deep, cracklike sores

cheiloschisis congenital cleft or split of the upper lip due to the failure of the maxillary bones (upper jaw) to fuse during embryonic development. Also known as *cleft lip* or *hare lip*.

chem/o chemical

chemotaxis migration of cells in response to a chemical stimulus. See **-taxis**.

chemotherapy use of chemical agents to treat disease. Today, chemotherapy has come to mean drugs used to treat cancer.

chest x-ray   X-ray images of the chest in the anteroposterior (AP), posteroanterior (PA), and/or lateral views without use of any contrast medium.

Chlamydia   A genus of microorganisms that causes a variety of diseases in humans.

chloride   See **mineral**.

cholangi/o bile duct; bile vessel

cholangiography process of producing an x-ray image of the bile ducts following intravenous injection of a contrast medium. Types include:

intravenous c. (IVC): contrast medium given by injection.
operative c.: contrast medium injected into the bile ducts at time of surgery
percutaneous transhepatic c.: contrast medium injected through the skin and liver into the biliary ducts
t-tube c.: contrast medium passed through a catheter shaped like a T

*chol*angio**pancreatography** process of producing an x-ray image of the bile ducts and pancreas following injection of a contrast medium

endoscopic retrograde cholangiopancreatography (ERCP): x-ray of the bile ducts and pancreas following placement of a contrast medium into the duodenum through an endoscope. Since the contrast medium flows backward into the pancreas from the duodenum, the term **retrograde**, meaning "to flow back," is used.

chol/e bile; gall

*chol*e**lith** a gallstone
*chol*e**lithiasis** abnormal condition of gallstones
*chol*e**stasis** stoppage of the flow of bile
*chol*e**sterol** a solid alcohol related to fats. Synthesized by the liver, cholesterol is a component of the plasma membrane. It is used to produce bile and steroid hormones (estrogen, progesterone, and testosterone); can accumulate and deposit abnormally, as in atherosclerosis or gallstones.

Memory Key: Cholesterol was first identified in gallstones, which were thought to be composed of solidified bile, hence the formation of the word cholesterol from **chol/e** (bile) + **stere/o** (solid) + **-ol** (alcohol).

*chol*e**steatoma** a cystlike mass of tissue in the middle ear obstructing the passage of sound waves. This is not a tumor in the normal sense, but an accumulation of cells forming a solid fatty mass. **Steat/o** means fat.

cholecyst/o gallbladder

*cholecyst*ectomy excision of the gallbladder
*cholecyst*itis inflammation of the gallbladder

cholecystogram record or image of the gallbladder produced by x-rays

cholecystokinin hormone secreted by the jejunum, duodenum, and hypothalamus. It stimulates the release of pancreatic juices and the contraction of the gallbladder.

Memory Key: The suffix **-in** refers to a chemical compound.

cholecystolithiasis abnormal condition of stones in the gallbladder; gallstones

choledoch/o common bile duct (CBD)

choledocholithiasis stones in the common bile duct

choledochotomy incision into the common bile duct

cholinergic fibers Nerve cell fibers that release acetylcholine as a neurotransmitter.

chondr/o cartilage

chondroblast immature cartilage cell

chondrocyte mature cartilage cell

chondrodysplasia inherited growth disorder of bone and cartilage leading to skeletal maldevelopment and dwarfism

chondroma benign tumor of cartilage

chondromalacia softening of cartilage

chondrosarcoma malignant tumor of cartilage

chordae tendineae Strong, tough cords that attach the flaps of the atrioventricular valves to the myocardium.

chori/o membrane

chorioretinitis inflammation of the choroid and retina

choroid thin, middle coat of the eye; vascular layer of the eye. (See Appendix F, Figure 15.)

choroid plexus network of capillaries in the brain. See **plexus**.

chorion The embryonic membrane that makes up part of the placenta.

chrom/o, chromat/o color

chromatin portion of the nucleus that contains DNA, carrier of the genes of inheritance. So named because it is readily stainable.

chromosome structure in the nucleus formed from chromatin. Chromosomes contain DNA that transmits genetic information.

hyperchromia a condition in which the red blood cells are darker than normal; red blood cells have increased pigmentation

hypochromia a condition in which the red blood cells are lighter in color than normal; red blood cells have decreased pigmentation

normochromia red blood cells that are of normal color

chronic
A disease characterized by gradual onset and long duration, for example, diabetes mellitus and osteoarthritis. Compare with **acute** and **subacute**.

Memory Key: Chron/o means "time"; a *chronic* disease persists over *time*.

chyle
Intestinal lymph.

chyme
A semisolid mixture of parcially digested food and gastric juices in the stomach.

chymotrypsin
An enzyme secreted by the pancreas that aids in the digestion of protein. **Chym/o** means "juice."

cicatrix
A scar.

cili/o hair

cilia hairlike processes projecting from certain cells, such as those in the bronchi or on the eyelids (eyelashes). Singular form is *cilium*.

ciliary body one of the structures of the eye making up the uvea. Consists of the ciliary processes and ciliary muscles.

ciliary muscles structure of the eye that adjusts the shape of the lens for focusing on objects

ciliary processes hairlike processes within the eye producing aqueous humor

supercilia eyebrows

circulatory system See **system**.

circum- around

circumcision removal of the prepuce or foreskin

circumduction process of drawing a structure, such as the arm or the leg, in a circular motion

circumvallate papillae circular projections at the back of the tongue containing taste buds. **Vallate** refers to "wall." Compare with **filiform** and **fungiform papillae**.

cirrhosis Chronic cellular degeneration of the liver. The most common cause of cirrhosis is alcoholism and is known as *Laënnec's cirrhosis*.

cis/o to cut

excision surgical removal of an organ or part by cutting

incision the process of cutting into a structure with a sharp instrument

citric acid cycle See **Krebs cycle**.

-clasis surgical fracture

osteoclasis surgical fracture or refracture of bone

-clast that which breaks down or destroys

osteoclasts bone cells that break down bone

claustrophobia Fear of enclosed places.

clavicle The collarbone. (See Appendix F, Figure 19.)

clavicul/o clavicle; collarbone

clavicular pertaining to the collarbone

cleft lip The congenital splitting of the upper lip. See **cheil/o, cheiloschisis**.

cleft palate The congenital splitting of the roof of the mouth. See **palat/o, palatoschisis**.

clitoris Portion of the female external genitalia analogous to the penis.

clonic contraction See **contraction**.

closed fracture A broken bone that does not pierce the skin; simple fracture.

clubfoot A congenital deformity of the foot. See **talipes**.

coagulation The process of clot formation.

coccyg/o tailbone; coccyx

coccygeal pertaining to the tailbone or coccyx

coccyx The tailbone. (See Appendix F, Figure 21.) See **vertebra**.

Memory Key: Coccyx comes from Greek *kokkyx* meaning "cuckoo bird." This name was given to the tailbone because it resembled the beak of a cuckoo.

cochle/o cochlea

Memory Key: Cochlea is Latin for "snail." The cochlea takes on a spiral formation resembling a snail shell.

cochlea one of several structures of the inner ear; resembles a snail shell. (See Appendix F, Figure 14.)
cochlear duct membranous duct inside the cochlea containing the main organ of hearing, the organ of Corti

coenzyme An inorganic substance associated with an enzyme that is required for the enzyme to function. For example, vitamins serve in many chemical reactions as coenzymes.

coitus Sexual intercourse.

collagen A glue-like protein substance found in skin, bone, tendons, and cartilage.

collateral ligaments Ligaments on the medial and lateral aspects of the knee joint providing stability for the knee. Included are the:

   lateral collateral l.: connects femur to fibula
   medial collateral l.: connects femur to tibia

collecting duct A component of the nephron attached to the distal convoluted tubule.

Colles' fracture A fracture of the distal radius. (See Appendix F, Figure 20.)

col/o, colon/o colon

colic condition usually seen in the first four months of life characterized by acute abdominal pain due to intestinal muscle spasms

colitis inflammation of the colon

colocolostomy creation of an anastomosis or new opening between two segments of the colon that were not previously together.

Memory Key: If the patient has advanced cancer of the ascending colon, which necessitates its entire removal, the transverse colon may be attached to the cecum. This new opening or connection between two segments of the colon is called *colocolostomy*.

colonoscopy process of viewing the colon with the aid of a colonoscope

colostomy creation of a new opening between the colon and the surface of the body.

colotomy process of cutting the colon

colon A segment of the large intestine. Includes the cecum, ascending colon, transverse colon, descending colon, and sigmoid colon. (See Appendix F, Figure 6.)

colostrum A nourishing fluid secreted from the mammary glands during the first few days following childbirth. The fluid contains antibodies to protect the infant.

colp/o vagina

colpoperineoplasty surgical reconstruction of the vagina and perineum

colporrhaphy suturing the vagina

colposcopy process of viewing the vagina with the aid of an instrument called a *colposcope*

coma A state of unconsciousness from which the patient cannot be roused.

comat/o deep sleep; coma

comatose pertaining to a coma

comminuted fracture A fracture in which the bone is splintered or crushed into several pieces. (See Appendix F, Figure 20.)

common bile duct (CBD) The duct of the digestion system leading into the duodenum; formed by the union of the hepatic and cystic ducts. Its function is to transport bile.

compact bone The dense, hard bone of the diaphysis of long bones.

complement A protein that **complements** the body's defense mechanism by assisting it in destroying invading microorganisms.

complete fracture A fracture in which the fracture line is continuous through the bone. (See Appendix F, Figure 20.)

compound fracture A fracture in which the broken bone pierces the skin; open fracture. (See Appendix F, Figure 20.)

concha Any structure that resembles a shell, such as the nasal conchae.

conduction system The electrical system of the heart that can function independently. Specialized muscle cells in the right atrium initiate electrical impulses that spread throughout the heart, causing it to contract. (See Appendix F, Figure 3.) Includes:

atrioventricular (AV) node: specialized cells at the base of the right atrium that receive electrical impulses from the sinoatrial (SA) node causing the atria to contract.

bundle branches: right and left branches of the bundle of His extending into the right and left ventricles. The fibers from each branch become continuous with the Purkinje fibers.

bundle of His (atrioventricular [AV] bundle): fibers that transmit electrical impulses through the heart originating from the atrioventricular node. The bundle of His divides into the right and left bundle branches.

Purkinje fibers: part of the conduction system of the heart that transmits impulses from the bundle branches into the ventricular endocardium; these fibers produce simultaneous contraction of the ventricles.

sinoatrial (SA) node or **pacemaker:** located in the right atrial wall, the SA node will initiate an electrical impulse simultaneously. It is called the *pacemaker* because it sets the heart's basic rhythm of 75 to 100 beats per minute.

condyle A bony projection that fits into a joint. This bony projection looks somewhat like a knuckle.

condyl/o knuckle

condyloma **acuminatum** a wart of viral origin located on the mucous membrane of the genital or anal areas. Associated with venereal disease.

Memory Key: Do not think that **condyloma** refers to a tumor of the bony condyle; rather, it is a growth on the mucous membrane that looks somewhat like a knuckle, hence its name.

cones Photoreceptors in the retina of the eye sensitive to bright light and color.

congenital Conditions that are present at birth. For example, a clubfoot or cleft palate.

congestive heart failure A condition in which myocardial disease results in the failure of the heart to pump blood effectively through the blood vessels, resulting in congestion of blood flow through the vascular system.

coni/o dust

pneumoconiosis abnormal accumulation of dust in the lungs. See **pneum/o, pneumoconiosis**.

conjunctiv/o conjunctiva

conjunctiva transparent membrane lining the eyelid and covering part of the eyeball. (See Appendix F, Figure 15.)

Memory Key: **-a** is a noun ending.

conjunctivitis inflammation of the conjunctiva; most common type is the acute contagious form also known as *pink eye*

connective tissue One of several types of tissue that functions to support and bind together the other tissues of the body.

contra- opposite; against

contraindication a term often used in pharmacology to refer to a disease or condition that makes the use of certain drugs harmful to the patient

***contra*lateral** pertaining to the opposite side

contraction The shortening or tightening of a muscle.

Braxton-Hicks c.: painless and irregular uterine contractions during pregnancy

clonic c.: alternating relaxation and contraction of a muscle in rapid succession.

isometric c.: contraction in which muscle length remains about the same while tension in the muscle increases.

isotonic c.: a contraction in which a muscle shortens while the tension in it remains the same. The shortening of the muscle during an isotonic contraction produces movement.

tonic c.: sustained muscle contraction in response to repetitive stimulation

contrast medium A substance that is placed in a patient's body before certain x-ray procedures. Some body parts are roughly the same density and, therefore, difficult to visualize. For this reason, radiologists order a contrast medium that will absorb x-rays at a different rate from the surrounding tissues, allowing clear visualization of the structure being examined. Barium is an example of a contrast medium.

convolution A bulge on the surface of the cerebral cortex; sulcus. (See Appendix F, Figure 11.)

corium The area of skin below the epidermis. Also known as *dermis*. (See Appendix F, Figure 22.)

corne/o cornea

cornea The transparent structure forming the outer layer of the eye. (See Appendix F, Figure 15.)

corneal reflex see **reflex**

corneal transplant see **kerat/o, keratoplasty**

coron/o crown

coronal plane See **plane, frontal plane**.

coronal suture See **suture**.

coronary arteries the arteries that supply the heart with blood

Memory Key: The coronary arteries sit on top of the heart like a crown.

coronary artery bypass graft (CABG) Surgery performed to reestablish adequate circulation to one or more segments of the heart when coronary artery disease diminishes blood flow

coronary circulation circulation of blood through the coronary arteries that supply the heart with blood.

corp/o body

corpus callosum bundle of nerve fibers connecting the right and left hemispheres of the brain allowing them to share information

corpus cavernosum erectile tissue of the penis and clitoris

corpus luteum a yellow body of cells that develops following the rupture of the graafian follicle (ovulation). The corpus luteum secretes progesterone and small amounts of estrogen.

corpus spongiosum erectile tissue in the penis

cortex The outer layer of any structure or organ, such as the adrenal cortex or cerebral cortex.

cortic/o cortex

adrenocorticotrophic hormone (ACTH) a hormone secreted by the pituitary gland to stimulate the release of hormones from the adrenal cortex. **-Trophic** means "nourishment."

corticosteroid hormones secreted by the adrenal cortex, such as cortisol, aldosterone, androgens, and estrogens

cost/o ribs

costochondral pertaining to the ribs and cartilage
costophrenic pertaining to the ribs and diaphragm
costosternal pertaining to the ribs and sternum
costovertebral pertaining to the ribs and vertebra

Cowper's gland The bulbourethral gland of the male reproductive system. See **gland, bulbourethral**. (See Appendix F, Figure 17.)

coxa valga The outward displacement of the hip joint. **Valga** means "bent outward."

coxa vara The inward displacement of the hip joint. **Vara** means "bent inward."

crani/o skull

cranium the skull, which includes the bony structures minus the lower jaw bone. (See Appendix F, Figure 19.)

Memory Key: Note the noun ending **-um**.

cranial bones skull bones including the frontal, parietal, temporal, occipital, sphenoid, ethmoid, nasal, vomer, and lacrimal bones, and the inferior nasal concha. (See Appendix F, Figure 19.)

Memory Key: Note the adjectival ending **-al**.

craniofacial pertaining to the head and face
craniometer instrument used to measure the skull
cranioplasty surgical reconstruction of the skull
craniotomy surgical incision into the skull

crepitus A grating or crackling sound heard on movement of ends of broken bones or in certain respiratory diseases. Also known as *crepitation*.

-crine secrete

apocrine gland type of exocrine gland that loses some of its cellular structure when secreting its product. **Apo-** means "derived from or away from." See **gland**.
eccrine gland secretes sweat. **Ec-** means "out." See **gland**.
endocrine gland secretes hormones directly into the blood stream. **Endo-** means "within." See **gland**.
exocrine gland secretes chemicals through ducts onto the surface of the skin or other organ. **Exo-** means "outside." See **gland**.

holocrine a type of exocrine gland in which the secretions contain entire secreting cells. **Hol/o** means "whole." See **gland**.

merocrine a type of exocrine gland in which the secretion of substances is through the plasma membrane. **Mer/o** means "part." See **gland**.

crin/o

endocrinology study of the diagnosis and treatment of disorders of the endocrine system

-crit derivative of -crine

hematocrit (HCT) a laboratory test that determines the percentage of erythrocytes in a blood sample

croup Inflammation of the larynx, trachea, and bronchus resulting in obstruction of the upper respiratory tract; laryngotracheobronchitis.

cruciate ligaments Cross-shaped ligaments supporting the knee joint between the femur and tibia.

cry/o cold

cryoprobe instrument used for the application of extreme cold to body tissues

cryotherapy treatment in which tissue is frozen, usually with liquid nitrogen; it is often used to destroy skin lesions such as warts

crypt/o hidden

cryptorchidism testicles that do not drop down into the scrotum from the abdomen during fetal development; undescended testicles

CT scan (computed tomography) A type of diagnostic procedure using x-rays. See **tom/o, tomography**.

cuboid   One of seven bones of the ankle. See **tarsal bones**.

cul-de-sac of Douglas   A pocket between the uterus and rectum. It is considered to be the lowest point in the abdominopelvic cavity, and as such, can be a gathering place for fluid and microorganisms. Also known as *rectouterine pouch* or *pouch of Douglas*. (See Appendix F, Figure 16.)

culd/o   Cul-de-sac (of Douglas).

*cul*docentesis   surgical puncture to remove fluid from the cul-de-sac of Douglas

*cul*doscopy   process of viewing the cul-de-sac of Douglas with the aid of a culdoscope

cuneiform   Three bones found at the ankle; 1st, 2nd, and 3rd cuneiforms. See **tarsal bones**.

-cuspid   points; projection; cusps

bi*cuspid*   having two points or projections

tri*cuspid*   having three points or projections

cutane/o

per*cutane*ous   pertaining to something done through the skin such as the injection of contrast medium or the application of sound waves

sub*cutane*ous   pertaining to under the skin; hypodermic

cyan/o   blue

*cyan*osis   abnormal bluish discoloration of the lips, skin, and mucous membrane due to the lack of oxygen in the blood

cyclic adenosine monophosphate (cAMP)   A substance that regulates the activities of a number of important enzymes.

cycl/o   ciliary body

*cycl*oplegia   paralysis of the ciliary body

cyclophotocoagulation destruction of a portion of the ciliary body using an intense beam of light from a laser

cyst A closed cavity or sac filled with a fluid, semifluid, or solid material. Types of cysts include:

follicular c.: involves the graafian follicle

lutein c.: involves the corpus luteum

ovarian c.: involves the ovary

sebaceous c.: involves the sebaceous glands

cyst/o sac; gallbladder; urinary bladder

cystic duct duct leading from the gallbladder

cystocele displacement of the urinary bladder against the wall of the vagina

cystourethrography x-ray of the urinary bladder and urethra following injection of a contrast medium in the bladder through a catheter. A *voiding cystourethrography* is an x-ray of the bladder and urethra while the patient is urinating

cystitis inflammation of the urinary bladder

cystoscopy process of viewing the urinary bladder with a cystoscope

cystostomy new opening into the urinary bladder for drainage

cystotomy incision into the urinary bladder

-cyte cell

adipocyte fat cell

chondrocyte a mature cartilage cell

erythrocyte a red blood cell

histiocyte a phagocytic cell present in connective tissue

leukocyte a mature white blood cell

osteocyte a mature bone cell

thrombocyte a cell responsible for clotting; platelet

cyt/o cell

cytology study of cells

cytochrome an important protein in cellular respiration responsible for electron transferring. Forms part of the electron transport chain.

cytokinesis the division of the cytoplasm into two parts occurring in the latter stages of mitosis

cytoplasm the portion of the cell between the cell membrane and nucleus. Contains the organelles.

cytoskeleton internal reinforcement of the cell, which is made up of microfilaments, microtubules, and intermediate filaments

cytosol the liquid portion within the cell membrane

cytotoxic T-lymphocytes white blood cells that kill body cells that have become infected by microorganisms; killer T-lymphocytes

cytotoxin an antibody that attacks the cells of a particular organ

-cytosis abnormal increase in the number of cells

erythrocytosis abnormal increase in the number of red blood cells

leukocytosis slight increase in the number of white blood cells caused by such conditions as fever, hemorrhage, infection, and inflammation

Memory Key: The use of the word *slight* is relative; in leukocytosis there is a slight increase in white blood cells when compared to leukemia in which there is a massive and malignant increase of white blood cells.

thrombocytosis abnormal increase in the number of thrombocytes in the blood

D

dacry/o tear

dacryoadenitis inflammation of the lacrimal gland

dacryocyst lacrimal sac

dacryocystitis inflammation of the lacrimal sac

dacryocystorhinostomy a new opening between the lacrimal sac and nose

dacryorrhea excessive flow of tears

dacryostenosis narrowing of the lacrimal duct

de- lack of; away from; down; not

débridement the removal of dead or damaged tissue and foreign material from an injured site

dedifferentiation loss of differentiation among cells. See **anaplasia**.

defecation evacuation of waste material from the digestive tract; expulsion of feces

Memory Key: Feces are the waste products from the digestive process combined with bacteria and cells.

defibrillation use of an electric shock to restore the heart to its normal rhythm when its contractions are irregular, uncoordinated, and of an extremely high number per minute; a clinical procedure that restores the heart to its normal rhythm following fibrillation. Also known as *cardioversion*.

deglutition swallowing

Memory Key: *Glutton* is a related word.

delirium a temporary mental condition characterized by confusion, excitement, and disorientation

Memory Key: The derivation of delirium is an interesting one. *Lira* is Latin for "groove or track." To the ancient Romans, if a person guiding a plow through a field strayed from the groove or track he was said to be delirious, hence a mentally confused person who could not plow a field. **Delirium** literally means "away from the groove."

delirium tremens (DTs) an acute delirious state caused by the withdrawal of alcohol, typically by alcoholics who have been drinking for many years

dementia a degeneration in mental and intellectual abilities. Literally means "out of mind."

demyelination degeneration of the myelin sheath covering a nerve fiber resulting in the failure of the nerve to transmit impulses. Characteristic of multiple sclerosis.

deoxygenated lack of oxygen. For example, the veins carry deoxygenated blood.

deoxyhemoglobin hemoglobin lacking oxygen

deoxyribonucleic acid (DNA) a nucleic acid containing the primary genetic material for living organisms

depolarization a change in the membrane potential in which the cell becomes positively charged in comparison to the charge outside the cell

desquamation shedding of skin; exfoliation. **Squam/o** means "scales."

decubitus Lying down.

decubitus ulcer An open sore caused by lying in one position for too long. See **ulcer**.

deep tendon reflexes See **reflex**.

decussate To cross from one side to the other in the form of an X. Usually refers to nerve cell fibers in the central nervous system.

dehiscence A splitting open, particularly of a healed wound or surgical incision.

delta wave A type of brain wave. See **wave**.

dendrite Tree-like projections from the cell body of a neuron that receive information from the internal and external environment.

dens A projection from the second cervical vertebra (C2) on which the head rotates. Also known as the *odontoid process*.

dense fibrous tissue A type of connective tissue.

dent/o tooth

dental caries tooth decay

dentin the entire tooth is surrounded by a hard bony layer of dentin that covers the softer pulp.

edentulous see **e-, edentulous**

deoxyribonucleic acid The carrier of genetic information. See **DNA**.

depression (1) A mark on a bone that is lower than the level of its surroundings. (2) An emotional state characterized by feelings of sadness, hopelessness, and despair.

-derm skin

ectoderm the outermost layer of embryonic germ cells that develops into the skin, nervous system, and outer structures of the eye and ear

endoderm the innermost layer of the embryonic germ cells that develops into the lining of tubes such as the respiratory and digestive tracts

mesoderm the middle germ layer of the embryo between the ectoderm and endoderm that develops into connective tissue such as muscles, skeletal structures, and blood vessels

dermat/o skin

dermatitis inflammation of the skin

dermatology branch of medicine dealing with the study of the diagnosis and treatment of skin disorders

dermatome (1) Instrument used to cut skin. (2) Specific areas of the skin stimulated by a single spinal nerve.

dermatomycosis fungal infection of the skin

dermatophytosis a fungal infection of the skin due to dermatophytes; causes such conditions as athlete's foot and jock itch

dermis
The layer of skin below the epidermis. Also known as *corium*. (See Appendix F, Figure 22.)

-desis surgical fusion

arthrodesis surgical fusion of a joint. See **arthr/o**.

dextrose
A monosaccharide also known as glucose.

di- two

diplegia paralysis affecting similar parts on both sides of the body, such as both arms or both legs

disaccharide a sugar composed of two monosaccharides

dia- through; completely; apart

diabetes insipidus the lack of or ineffectiveness of the anti-diuretic hormone (ADH), resulting in excessive urination

Memory Key: Because of the excessive volume of water in the urine, the urine is tasteless or insipid.

diabetes mellitus impaired insulin secretion and/or effective-ness that results in improper metabolism of carbohydrates, fats, and proteins

Memory Key: Diabetes means "running through," which relates to excessive urination, one of the chief symptoms of diabetes. **Mellitus** means "sweetened with honey," referring to the sweetness of urine due to the elevated sugar.

diagnosis one disease is differentiated from another disease after complete knowledge is obtained of the disease through a study of the signs, symptoms, and laboratory, x-ray, and other diagnostic procedures

dialysis mechanical replacement of kidney function when the kidney is dysfunctional

diapedesis passage of blood cells into tissues through an intact blood vessel wall

diaphoresis A state of profuse sweating. **Phoresis** means "transmission; carry."

diaphragm A respiratory muscle separating the thoracic and abdominal cavities. **Phragm** means "wall." (See Appendix F, Figure 18.)

diaphysis shaft of a long bone

diarrhea bowel movements that are too frequent and loose

diastole dilatation of the myocardium during the cardiac cycle. In **atrial diastole**, the atria dilate and fill with blood; in **ventricular diastole**, the ventricles dilate and fill with blood. Diastole of the ventricles occurs after that of the atria. Compare with **systole**. **Stole** means "put; place."

diastolic pressure Pressure against the wall of an artery during diastole, when the ventricles are relaxed.

diathermy heat applied to deep tissues

differentiated
A term used to describe normal cells in which similar cells are capable of performing their own function, which varies from that of other cells. Compare with **dedifferentiated** under **de-**.

diffusion
The spontaneous movement of molecules from an area of higher to lower concentration.

digestion
The breaking down of food into chemical substances to be utilized by the body.

digestive system
See **system**.

digital subtraction angiography
An x-ray of the blood vessels. See **angiography**.

diplo- double

diplococcus gram-positive spherical bacteria occurring in pairs

diploid human cells possessing 46 chromosomes

diplopia double vision

-dipsia thirst

oligodipsia diminished thirst

polydipsia excessive thirst

dis- away from; separation; apart

dislocation displacement of a joint structure from its original position. May be a partial or complete dislocation.

dissect to cut and separate body tissues and parts for study

dissecting aneurysm abnormal dilatation of an artery in which the blood seeps between the layers of the arterial wall

disc A flat, circular, platelike structure. Also spelled *disk*.

disease A pathological state manifested by a group of signs and symptoms that deviates from the normal structure and function of the body organs.

distal Farthest away from the point of origin of a body part or farthest away from the point of attachment of the arm to the trunk. Opposite is *proximal*.

Memory Key: The intestines are *distal* to the stomach as the mouth is the point of origin. The wrist is *distal* to the elbow as the wrist is farther away from the point of attachment to the trunk.

diuresis Increased urination.

diverticulitis Inflamed diverticulum.

diverticulum An outpouching of the walls of the large intestine. Debris may become trapped in the pouch causing an inflammation called diverticulitis. Plural is *diverticula*.

Memory Key: Diverticulum literally means "turns aside." Think of this abnormal pouch turning away from the normal alignment of the intestine, forming a separate channel or pouch.

DNA

A nucleic acid containing the elements of oxygen, carbon, hydrogen, phosphorous, and nitrogen. DNA contains the cell basis of heredity and is the carrier of genetic information. Abbreviation for deoxyribonucleic acid.

donor

One who donates.

dopamine

A neurotransmitter; a catecholamine produced in the adrenal gland that acts to increase blood pressure.

dorsi-, dors/o back

dorsal cavity hollow space located at the back of the body divided into the cranial cavity containing the brain and the spinal cavity containing the spine

dorsal column white matter of the spinal cord. See **poster/o, posterior column**.

dorsal horn gray matter of the spinal cord. See **poster/o, posterior horn**.

dorsalis pedis pulse pulse point that can be felt on the dorsum of the foot

Memory Key: *Dorsum* refers to the upper convex portion of the foot.

dorsal recumbent lying down on the back

dorsal root attaches a spinal nerve to the spinal cord. See **poster/o, posterior root**.

dorsiflexion joint movement bending the part toward the dorsum or upper convex portion. For example, dorsiflexion at the ankle moves the foot toward the shin; dorsiflexion at the wrist moves the hand backward toward the elbow.

-drome to run

prodrome symptoms occurring before the onset of disease. See **pro-, prodrome**.

syndrome signs and symptoms occurring (running) together and indicating a particular condition or disease

duct/o draw; lead

ab*duction* process of drawing a part, such as the arms or legs, away from the midline

ad*duction* process of drawing a part, such as the arms or legs, toward the midline

circum*duction* process of drawing a part, such as the arm, in a circular motion

ductus deferens Vas deferens; structure of the male reproductive system that transports sperm. (See Appendix F, Figure 17.)

duoden/o duodenum

*duoden***ocholangitis** inflammation of the duodenum and common bile duct

*duoden***ojejunostomy** new opening (anastomosis) between the duodenum and jejunum

*duoden***orrhaphy** suturing of the duodenum

*duoden***um** first segment of the small intestine. (See Appendix F, Figure 6.)

dur/o tough

*dur***a mater** the outermost membrane of the brain and spinal cord. Also known as *pachymeninges*. See **mening/o, meninges**. (See Appendix F, Figure 12.)

dynia pain

arthro*dynia* joint pain

gastrox*dynia* stomach pain

dys- bad; painful; difficult

*dys***arthria** difficulty in articulating speech due to muscular incoordination resulting from nerve damage

*dys***chromia** abnormal color of skin

*dys***entery** refers to any number of painful intestinal disorders

*dys***esthesia** an irritating sensation in response to normal stimuli

*dys***kinesia** impaired muscle movement

*dys***menorrhea** painful menstruation

dyspareunia painful sexual intercourse

Memory Key: Pareunia means "lying beside."

dyspepsia indigestion

dysphagia difficulty in swallowing

dysphasia impairment of speaking usually due to brain dysfunction

dysphonia difficulty in speaking; hoarseness

dysplasia abnormal development of tissue

dyspnea difficulty in breathing

dysrhythmia disturbance in the rhythm of the heart or speech

dysthymia mood disorder characterized by a feeling of sadness and a loss of pleasure or interest in daily activities; however, not severe enough to be classified as a major depression

dystocia difficult labor

dystonia abnormal muscle tone often resulting in abnormal muscle movement

dystrophy abnormal growth or development

dysuria painful urination

E

e- out; outward

edentulous without teeth

eversion turning of the sole of the foot outward away from the midline

eardrum The tympanic membrane. (See Appendix F, Figure 14.)

ec- out; out of

ecchymosis large, purplish, subcutaneous spot caused by hemorrhaging into the skin. Also known as a bruise. Compare with **petechia**.

eccrine gland type of sweat gland. See **gland**.

ectopic out of place. For example, in an ectopic pregnancy the fetus matures in a place other than the uterus such as the fallopian tube.

ectropion outward turning of the eyelid

ECG, EKG, electrocardiogram See **electr/o, electrocardiogram**.

ech/o sound

echocardiogram the record or image of the heart produced by high frequency sound waves. See **ultrasound** definition (2).

echocardiography process of obtaining an image of the anatomical structures of the heart and of the blood flow through the cardiovascular system by using high frequency sound waves. Also measures strength of left ventricular contraction.

echoencephalography process of producing an image of the brain using high frequency sound waves. See **ultrasound** definition (2).

echogenic body tissues giving rise to echoes of ultrasound

echogram see **ultrasonogram**

echography the process of using high frequency sound waves to produce an image. See **ultrasound** definition (2).

-ectasis dilatation; dilation

angiectasis dilatation of a blood vessel

atelectasis incomplete expansion of the alveoli of the lung

bronchiectasis abnormal widening or dilatation of the bronchi

ecto- outside

ectoderm outer layer of embryonic cells. See **-derm**.

ectogenous produced from outside of the body; disease that originates from outside the body. Also known as *exogenous*; opposite is *endogenous*.

-ectomy excision; surgical removal

Memory Key: **-ectomy** is a common suffix formed by **ec-** meaning "out" and **-tomy** meaning "to cut." **-ectomy** preceded by an anatomical root means the surgical removal of that anatomical structure.

gastrectomy surgical removal of the stomach
hysterectomy surgical removal of the uterus
tonsillectomy surgical removal of the tonsils

eczema A superficial skin condition characterized by itching, redness, and inflammation; cause unknown.

edema The accumulation of excess fluid in tissue spaces.

effector An organ or muscle that responds to a stimulus.

efferent To carry away from. See **ex-, efferent**.

effusion To pour out. See **ex-, effusion**.

ejaculatory duct The extension of the vas deferens as it joins the urethra. (See Appendix F, Figure 17.)

elasticity The ability of tissue to return to its normal size and shape after stretching.

elastin A protein substance forming the primary constituent of elastic tissue.

electr/o electric

*electro*cardiogram **(ECG, EKG)** record of the electrical activity of the heart, recorded as waves. Different wave forms are produced by different portions of the cardiac cycle: **P wave** (atrial contraction), **QRS wave** (ventricular contraction), and **T wave** (ventricular relaxation).
*electro*cardiograph instrument used to record the electrical activity of the heart
*electro*cochleography process of recording the electrical activities of the cochlea

***electro*encephalogram (EEG)** record of the electrical activity of the brain measured in waves of activity. Included are **alpha waves** typical of an awake person at rest, **beta waves** typical of increased neural activity, **delta waves** typical of deep sleep, and **theta waves** most often seen in children but may occur in adults under emotional stress.

***electro*encephalograph** instrument used to record the electrical activity of the brain

***electro*lysis** destruction of tissue by electricity

***electro*lyte** a solute capable of conducting an electric current

***electro*myogram** record of the electrical activity of a muscle

***electro*n** a minute, negatively charged particle that moves rapidly around the nucleus of an atom

***electro*phoresis** a laboratory test in which substances in a mixture, usually proteins, are separated by an electrical current

element
A substance that cannot be decomposed by chemical means. For example: oxygen, hydrogen, nitrogen, calcium, and phosphorus.

elevation
The movement of body parts to a point of greater height.

embolus
A blood clot or foreign clump of material moving through a blood vessel. See **bol-**.

embryo
The name given to the human organism from the third week to the end of the eighth week of development. Compare with **fetus**.

-emesis vomiting
hemat*emesis* vomiting of blood

melan*emesis* black vomit. See **melan/o, melanemesis**

hyper*emesis* excessive vomiting

hyper*emesis* gravidarum excessive vomiting during pregnancy

emetic
An agent that induces vomiting.

-emia blood condition

anemia lack of red blood cells. See **a(n), anemia**.
hyperglycemia excessive blood sugar
ischemia holding back of blood to a part. See **isch/o, ischemia**
polycythemia increase in the total number of red blood cells
septicemia the presence of disease causing microorganisms in the blood

emmetropia Normal vision.

emphysema The over-inflation of the air sacs of the lung with associated destruction of the alveolar walls, resulting in extremely difficult breathing.

empyema Pus in the pleural cavity; pyothorax.

emulsification The process of breaking down large fat droplets into smaller fat droplets.

enamel The hard, thin, calcified substance that covers the crown of the tooth.

encephal/o brain

encephalitis inflammation of the brain
encephalocele hernia of the brain and meninges; protrusion of the brain and meninges through a defect in the skull
encephalomalacia softening of the brain
encephalopathy any disease of the brain

endo- within; innermost

endarterectomy removal of the inner lining of the arterial wall. A surgical procedure to treat atherosclerosis.
endocarditis inflammation of the inner lining of the heart
endocardium innermost layer of the heart. Compare with **epicardium**, **myocardium**, and **pericardium**.
endocrine gland see **gland**
endocrine system see **system**
endocrinologist specialist in the study of the endocrine glands and the diagnosis and treatment of their disorders
endoderm inner layer of embryonic cells. See **-derm**.

endodontist dentist who specializes in the diagnosis and treatment of diseases within the tooth, such as the pulp

endogenous disease that originates from inside the body. Opposite is **ectogenous**

endolymph a fluid within the membranous labyrinth of the inner ear. Compare with **perilymph**.

endometriosis endometrial tissue found at sites other than the uterus

endometrium inner lining of the uterus. The superficial layers of the endometrium are sloughed off during menstruation.

endomysium a sheath of connective tissue that surrounds each muscle fiber. Compare with **epimysium** and **perimysium**.

endoplasmic reticulum microscopic channels or tubes extending throughout the cytoplasm; serves as a transport system for materials within the cell

endoscope a fiber-optic instrument used to visually examine a body cavity or organ. It can be inserted through a body cavity or through a small incision. Endoscopes are named after the organ being examined. For example: a gastroscope visually examines the stomach, a colonoscope visually examines the colon.

endoscopic retrograde cholangiopancreatography (ERCP) process of recording the bile ducts and pancreas using x-rays. See **ERCP** under **cholangi/o**.

endosteum connective tissue lining the medullary cavity of a long bone

endothelium type of epithelial tissue. See **thel/o**.

endotoxin poisonous substance in bacteria. See **tox/o, endotoxin**

endotracheal intubation procedure in which a flexible tube is inserted through the nose or mouth, and then pushed through the pharynx, larynx, and into the trachea to establish an airway

end-plate potential The electrical stimulation of a muscle fiber that results from the release of neurotransmitters causing sodium ions to enter the muscle fiber.

energy The ability to do work.

enter/o intestine, often small intestine

enteritis inflammation of the small intestine
enterocolitis inflammation of the small intestine and colon
enterogastric pertaining to the intestine and stomach
enterotomy incision into the small intestine

entropion The inward turning of the eyelid.

enzyme A protein substance that is a catalyst for chemical reactions.

eosinophil A type of white blood cell. See **-phil**.

epi- upon; on; above

epicardium outermost layer of the heart. Also known as the visceral pericardium. Compare with **myocardium**, **endocardium**, and **pericardium**.
epicondyle bony projection above or on top of a condyle. See **condyle**.
epidermis outermost layer of the skin located above the dermis. The epidermis itself has five thin layers of epithelial tissue. (See Appendix F, Figure 22.)
epididymis coiled tube on the superior surface of each testicle. The epididymis stores sperm and leads into the vas deferens. **-didymis** refers to the paired testicles. (See Appendix F, Figure 17.)
epidural pertaining to upon or outside the dura mater
epidural anesthesia injection of a local anesthetic into the epidural space around the spinal cord to provide anesthesia to the genital or pelvic areas
epidural space area above the dura mater of the brain and spinal cord
epigastrium area of the abdomen located above the umbilicus. Compare with **hypogastrium** under **hypo-**.

Memory Key: In this case **gastr/o** means "belly," referring to the umbilicus.

epiglottis a lidlike structure that covers the opening of the larynx during swallowing, thereby sealing the air passage

epilepsy seizure disorder due to uncoordinated and disorganized electrical impulses in the brain. See **seizure**.

Memory Key: Epilepsy means "to seize upon"; the patient having the seizure was thought to be seized by an unknown influence.

epimysium connective tissue that forms the outermost covering of the skeletal muscle. Compare with **endomysium** and **perimysium**.

epinephrine (1) Hormone secreted by the adrenal medulla. Also known as *adrenaline*. (2) Neurotransmitter secreted by some neurons.

Memory Key: Epi- means "upon," **nephr/o** means "kidney," **-ine** means "chemical." Epinephrine is a chemical secreted by the adrenal medulla, which sits upon the kidney.

epiphyseal line the name given to the epiphyseal plate when the bone has stopped growing

epiphyseal plate cartilage that divides the diaphysis from the epiphysis in a growing bone. Also known as *epiphyseal cartilage*. The epiphyseal plate gives way to the epiphyseal line when the bone stops growing.

epiphysis bulbous portion at the proximal and distal ends of the long bone

epispadias congenital defect in which the urethral meatus is located on the dorsum (top side) of the penis. Compare with **hypospadias** under **hypo-**.

epithelium epithelial tissue. See **thel/o**.

eponychium cuticle; literally means "structure upon the nail"

Memory Key: Note that the **i** in **epi-** is dropped as the root starts with a vowel.

episi/o external genitalia; vulva

episiorrhaphy suturing of the vulva and perineum, usually at the time of delivery, to repair lacerations that may occur as the head of the fetus is being delivered through the birth canal

episiotomy incision of the vulva, especially in the area between the vagina and anus, to assist in delivery of the fetus

epistaxis A nose bleed; rhinorrhagia.

erythema A red discoloration of the skin.

erythr/o red

erythremia abnormal increase in the number of red blood cells. Also known as *polycythemia vera*.

erythroblast immature red blood cell

erythroblastosis fetalis destruction of red blood cells in the newborn due to Rh incompatibility between the mother and fetus. Also known as hemolytic disease of the newborn.

erythrocyte mature red blood cell

erythrocytopenia deficiency of red blood cells; erythropenia

erythrocytosis increase in the number of red blood cells

erythropenia See **erythrocytopenia**.

erythropoiesis production of red blood cells

erythropoietin a hormone in the kidney which stimulates the production of red blood cells

esotropia Inward turning of the eyeball; strabismus.

-esthesia sensation

anesthesia loss of sensation. See **a(n), anesthesia**.

dysesthesia an irritating sensation in response to normal stimuli

hyperesthesia increased or exaggerated sensations, particularly a painful sensation from a normally painless touch

hypoesthesia decreased sensations particularly to touch

paresthesia abnormal sensation such as numbness and tingling often occurring without external stimulation. **Para-** means "abnormal."

Memory Key: Note the final vowel is dropped in **para-** because the suffix begins with a vowel.

estrogens A group of hormones secreted by the ovaries, placenta, and in small amounts by the testes and adrenal cortex. Estrogen is responsible for many female reproductive functions including secondary female characteristics and is used in the treatment of some male reproductive cancers.

ethmoid bone One of the bones of the skull.

Memory Key: Ethm/o means "sieve-like." Portions of the ethmoid bone have tiny holes resembling a sieve.

eu- good

euphoria an exaggerated feeling of well-being

eupnea normal, regular breathing

euthanasia death with little or no pain. Euthanasia involves the administration of a drug in large enough quantities to end the suffering of an incurable disease and painful death. Also known as *mercy killing*.

euthyroid thyroid that functions properly

eutocia normal labor

eustachian tube Tube leading from the throat to

the middle ear. Also known as *auditory tube*. (See Appendix F, Figure 14.)

ex- out; outside

efferent to carry away from the center. For example, efferent arteries carry blood away from the heart and efferent neurons carry electrical impulses away from the brain and spinal cord.

Memory Key: Ex- changes to **ef-** before suffixes that begin with **f**; however, there are some exceptions as in *exfoliation*.

effusion an abnormal accumulation of fluid into a part or tissue; a pouring out. See Memory Key under **ex, efferent**.

excision process of cutting out, such as the removal of an organ by cutting

excoriation scratch or abrasion of the skin

Memory Key: Cori refers to **corium**, the deeper layer of skin.

excretion the separation or movement of substances outward, from the internal to the external environment

excretory urogram x-ray of the urinary system. See **ur/o, urogram**.

exfoliation shedding, scaling, or desquamation of epidermal cells

expiration to breathe out

expiratory reserve volume (ERV) see **pulmon/o, pulmonary function test**

exacerbation a worsening of symptoms. Opposite is **remission**

exo- out; outside

exocrine gland secretes chemicals through ducts outward onto the surface of an organ. See **gland**.

exogenous see **ectogenous**

exophthalmos outward protrusion of the eyeball

exotoxin poisonous substance secreted by living bacterial cells

exotropia outward turning of the eyeball; strabismus

extension Return from flexion; increasing the angle between two bones; straightening out a limb.

external auditory meatus The bilateral tubes that transmit sound waves from the external to middle ear. (See Appendix F, Figure 14.)

external respiration See **respiration**.

extra- out; outside

extracellular fluid body fluids located outside the cell, including the interstitial fluid and plasma

extracorporeal circulation circulation of blood outside the body. For example, the circulation of blood through a heart-lung machine for oxygen-carbon dioxide exchange during surgical procedures.

extraocular outside the eyeball

extravasation the escape of fluid, such as blood, from a blood vessel

exudate The passing out of fluid from a vessel wall into a cavity or neighboring tissue, usually as a result of inflammation.

F

facet A small, smooth joint surface on a bone.

fallopian tube A structure of the female reproductive system that carries the egg or ova from the ovary to the uterus. Also known as *uterine tubes* or *oviducts*. (See Appendix F, Figure 11.)

false ribs See **ribs.**

false vocal cords Cords in the larynx that do not produce sounds.

farsightedness A vision defect resulting in sharp focus only for objects far from the eye. See **hyper-, hypermetropia**.

fasciculation An uncontrollable, localized contraction of a single muscle group visible through the skin.

fasciculus A small bundle of nerves, muscles, or tendon fibers.

fasci/o fascia

fascia a band of connective tissue lying deep in the skin and enveloping muscles and other body organs

fasciectomy excision of the fascia

fasciitis; *fascitis* inflammation of the fascia

fasciorrhaphy suturing of the fascia

fat
White or yellowish adipose tissue forming a cushioning layer between organs and providing a source of energy for the body.

fatigue, muscle
A condition in which repeated stimulation over an extended period of time makes the muscle unable to contract.

fatty acid
An end product of fat digestion in which triglycerides are broken down into fatty acids and glycerol; may be **saturated**, having single bonds, or **unsaturated**, having double or triple bonds.

febrile
Feverish; having a fever.

feces
Waste products excreted from the intestines consisting of bacteria, intestinal secretions, cells, and a small amount of food residue.

femor/o femur; thigh bone

femoral pertaining to the femur

femoral canal a tubular channel for the passage of blood vessels and nerves to the thigh

femoral hernia see **hernia**

femoroiliac pertaining to the femur and ilium (hip)

femur
The long bone extending from the pelvis to the knee; thigh bone. (See Appendix F, Figure 19.)

fertilization
The union of the ovum and sperm, usually occurring in the fallopian tube.

fetal alcohol syndrome (FAS) A group of
congenital defects occurring in infants born of mothers who
chronically consumed alcohol during pregnancy.

fet/o fetus

fetus a developing organism from the end of its eighth week
of development until birth

Memory Key: -us is a noun suffix meaning "a thing."

fetometry process of measuring the fetus, particularly the
diameter of its head

fetoscope instrument used to visually examine the fetus while
in the uterus

fibrillation, ventricular Abnormal rhythm of
the heart characterized by an extremely high number of
irregular, uncoordinated ventricular contractions.

fibrinogen A plasma protein necessary for blood
clotting.

fibr/o fibers or fibrous tissue

fibrin a protein whose fibers entangle blood cells, the whole
forming a blood clot

Memory Key: -in means "chemical compound."

fibroadenoma benign glandular tumor containing fibrous
tissue, often occurring in the breasts

fibroblast a connective tissue cell that develops into many
of the cells that form the fibrous tissue in the body such
as tendons, ligaments, and aponeuroses. Also known as a
fibrocyte.

fibrocartilaginous pertaining to fibrous and cartilaginous
tissue

Memory Key: Note that the **e** in **cartilage** is changed to
an **i** in **cartilaginous**

fibrocyte see **fibroblast**

fibroid resembling anything that has a fibrous structure; often used to mean a fibroma

fibroma benign tumor composed mainly of fibrous connective tissue often occurring in the uterus; a leiomyoma

fibromyalgia pain of fibrous tissues such as muscles, tendons, and ligaments

fibromyoma benign tumor of the smooth muscle tissue of the uterus

fibul/o fibula

fibula small bone of the lower leg attached laterally to the tibia. (See Appendix F, Figure 19.)

Memory Key 1: Fibula is Latin for "clasp" or "pin;" the fibula is pinned to the tibia like a brooch.

Memory Key 2:: -a is the noun ending.

filiform papillae The rough surface at the front of the tongue that aids in licking. Compare with **circumvallate** and **fungiform** papillae.

filtrate Fluid that a filter allows to pass through.

fimbria Fingerlike projections extending from the distal ends of the fallopian tubes.

fissure A narrow, deep, slitlike opening. May be anatomical as in the fissures of the brain or pathological as in anal fissure, which is a cracklike sore of the mucous membrane of the anus.

fistula Abnormal passage between two internal organs or between an organ and the surface of the body.

Memory Key: Fistula is Latin for "water pipe" or "tube."

flaccid Having no muscle tone.

flagellum Hairlike projections extending from the surface of a cell such as a sperm cell; aids in the movement of sperm cells.

flatulence   The presence of gas or air in the digestive tract causing distention of the organ. **Flatus** is the gas or air that is expelled.

Memory Key: In*flate*, de*flate*, and *flute* all contain the same Latin root.

flexion   A movement that decreases the angle at a joint.

flexors   Muscles that bend a joint.

floating ribs   See **ribs**.

fluoroscopy   X-ray examination of a structure to include not only its size and shape, but also its movements, such as the movement of substances through the digestive tract. Fluoroscopy has the advantage of revealing subtle changes in anatomic structures that may obstruct the normal passage of intestinal contents. Fluoroscopy is used in barium studies and to guide the insertion of catheters.

Foley catheter   A flexible tube inserted through the urethra into the urinary bladder to drain urine.

follicle   An anatomical structure resembling a sac or bag. Various types of follicles include:

graafian f.: a cell mass containing the developed ovum
hair f.: sac from which a hair grows
ovarian f.: sac containing the ovum at any stage of development
thyroid f.: a spherical structure in the thyroid gland that secretes the thyroid hormone

fontanel, fontanelle   The soft spot lying between the cranial bones of the fetus or infant.

foramen   A hole or opening. Examples include:

f. magnum: large opening in the occipital bone for the passage of the spinal cord

f. ovale: opening in the fetal heart for the passage of blood from the right to the left atrium

nutrient f.: opening in a bone for the passage of blood vessels and nerves

obturator f.: large opening in the pelvic bone, between the ischium and pubis, for the passage of blood vessels and nerves to the thigh

forebrain The largest division of the brain consisting of the cerebrum, thalamus, and hypothalamus.

foreskin The skin covering the tip of the penis

fornix An arch-shaped roof of an anatomical space. Fornices are present in the vagina, conjunctivae, brain, and pharynx.

fossa A depression in a body structure.

fovea centralis A structure of the eye located in the center of the macula lutea of the retina that contains the cones, making it the area of clearest vision.

fracture A break in a bone; discontinuity in the normal alignment of bone. (See Appendix F, Figure 20.) Types of fractures include:

closed f.: the broken bone does not pierce the skin. Also known as *simple f.*

Colles' f.: break of the distal radius.

comminuted f.: bone is crushed or splintered.

complete f.: fracture line is continuous through the bone.

compound f.: bone pierces the skin. Also known as *open f.*

greenstick f.: a type of partial fracture, which like a green stick or twig from a tree, will bend on one side and break on the other.

impacted f.: the fracture is caused by the impact of one bone hitting another.

incomplete f.: fracture line is not continuous through the bone. Also known as *partial f.*

intra-articular f.: the fracture line is on the joint surfaces of bone.

linear f.: the fracture line runs parallel to the axis of the bone.

open f.: see *compound f.*

partial f.: see *incomplete f.*

Pott's f.: a break in the distal fibula and medial malleolus.

simple f.: see *closed f.*

spiral f.: the fracture line curves around the bone.

stellate f.: the fracture lines radiate from a specific point of injury.

stress f.: a slight disruption in the bone due to continuous impacts, such as those caused by jumping or running.

transverse f.: the fracture line runs across the bone at right angles to its axis.

free radical
A molecule containing an odd number of electrons.

fremitus
Vibrations felt through the chest wall as the patient makes vocal sounds.

frenulum
The tough fibrous cord connecting the tongue to the floor of the mouth.

front/o front

frontal **bone** cranial bone forming the forehead and the superior portion of the orbits. (See Appendix F, Figure 19.)

frontal **lobe** front portion of the cerebrum. See **lob/o** for a complete listing of lobes. (See Appendix F, Figure 11.)

frontal **plane** see **plane**

fructose
A monosaccharide found in fruit juices and honey; a simple sugar.

fulguration The destruction of unwanted tissue by the use of electrical energy in the form of sparks.

fundus The base or bottom of an anatomical structure usually farthest away from its opening. For example:

f. of the eye: part farthest away from the cornea; back portion of the eye

f. of the stomach: part farthest away from the pyloric sphincter. (In this example, the opening is the pyloric sphincter rather than the gastroesophageal sphincter.)

f. of the uterus: part farthest away from the cervix

funduscopy The process of visually examining the eye. Also known as *ophthalmoscopy*.

Memory Key: In the term *fund**u**scopy*, the combining vowel **u** is used instead of **o**.

fungiform papillae The small rounded projections on the middle and anterior segments of the tongue containing taste buds. Compare with **filiform** and **circumvallate papillae**.

furuncle A boil.

G

GABA Gamma-aminobutyric acid.

gag reflex See **reflex**.

galact/o milk

Memory Key: Relate **galact/o** to *galaxy*, as in the Milky Way.

***galacto*cele** protrusion or swelling caused by the accumulation of milk in a blocked milk duct of the breast

***galacto*rrhea** discharge of milk from the breast at a time other than nursing a newborn or infant; excessive discharge of milk from the breast

***galacto*se** a monosaccharide or simple sugar found in lactose

gallbladder
A pear-shaped structure located under the liver in the right upper quadrant of the abdomen; functions to store bile. (See Appendix F, Figure 6.)

gallium 67 (^{67}Ga)
A radioisotope utilized in the scanning of neoplasms, inflammation, and soft tissue. See **radi/o, radioisotope**.

gallstone
The accumulation of cholesterol and a variety of bile components forms into a hard stone or calculus, which may block the passage of bile as it travels from the gallbladder into the duodenum.

gamete
A mature reproductive cell. The male gametes are spermatozoa, the female gametes are ova.

gamma-aminobutyric acid
A neurotransmitter in the brain.

gamma globulin
A grouping of plasma proteins to which most of the immune antibodies belong. Also known as *immunoglobulins* (Ig). Divided into five classes: IgA, IgD, IgE, IgG, and IgM.

ganglion
(1) Anatomical meaning: a group of nerve cell bodies located outside the brain and spinal cord. Ganglions act as relay stations receiving, organizing, and sending impulses throughout the body. (2) Pathological meaning: a cystic mass arising from a tendon sheath frequently occurring on the wrist.

gastr/o   stomach

gastralgia   stomachache; gastrodynia

gastrectomy   excision of the stomach

gastric juice   accumulation of gastric secretions, such as mucus, hydrochloric acid, intrinsic factor, and pepsinogen

gastric lavage   to wash out or irrigate the stomach; to pump the stomach of toxic contents. Compare with **gastrogavage** under **gastr/o**.

Memory Key: Lavage means "washing." Related term is **lav**atory.

gastrin   hormone secreted by the stomach

gastritis   inflammation of the stomach

gastrocolostomy   new opening between the stomach and large intestine. The surgical joining of two structures that are normally separate is called *anastomosis*. See **ana, anastomosis**.

gastrodynia   stomachache; gastralgia

gastroenteritis   inflammation of the stomach and intestines

gastroenterologist   specialist in the diagnosis and treatment of disorders of the stomach and intestines

gastroesophageal reflux   backward flow of gastric contents into the esophagus. Also known as *heartburn*.

gastrogavage   passage of a tube into the stomach for the provision of nutrients when the patient cannot take food in the conventional manner; forced feeding. Compare with **gastric lavage** under **gastr/o**.

Memory Key: Gavage means "stuffing."

gastrointestinal tract (GIT)   a hollow tube extending from the mouth to the anus. Also known as the *digestive tract* and *alimentary tract*.

gastrojejunostomy   new opening between the stomach and jejunum. The surgical joining of two structures that are normally separate is called *anastomosis*. See **ana-, anastomosis**.

gastrorrhagia   bleeding from the stomach

gastrorrhaphy   suturing or sewing of a wound in the stomach wall

gastrostomy   creation of a new opening into the stomach

gastrotomy process of cutting the stomach

gastrocnemius The calf muscle at the back of the leg.

Memory Key: Are you wondering why the root **gastr/o** appears in this word? **Gastr/o** originally meant "belly;" **cnemius** means "leg," hence muscle belly of the leg.

gene The basic unit of heredity occupying a certain location on a chromosome. Genes are composed of DNA.

generalized seizure See **seizure**.

-genic producing
carcinogenic agent that produces cancer

genitalia The internal and external organs associated with reproduction; includes both male and female organs.

genital herpes An infection of the skin and mucous membrane of the genitals, usually caused by the microorganism herpes simplex virus type II, although it may also be caused by herpes simplex virus type I.

genotype The genetic makeup of an individual.

-genous producing
ectogenous; exogenous produced from outside the body; disease that originates outside the body
endogenous produced from inside the body; disease that originates from inside the body

genu knee
Memory Key: A related term is **genuflect** meaning "a bending at the knees."

***genu* valgum** knock-kneed; legs bent inward at the knee. See **valgus**; **genu valgum**.

genu **varum** bow-legged; legs bent outward at the knee. See **varus**; **genu varum**.

geri-, geront/o old age

geriatrics branch of medicine dealing with the treatment of problems particular to old age

gerontology the study of the problems particular to old age

Gerota's fascia Connective tissue surrounding and supporting the kidney; renal fascia.

gestation The length of time the developing organism is in utero from conception to birth.

gingiv/o gums

gingivitis inflammation of the gums

gingivobuccal pertaining to the gums and cheek

gingivoglossitis inflammation of the gums and tongue

gland An organ whose main function is the production and secretion of certain substances.

adrenal g.: located on top of each kidney. Adrenal **cortex** is the outer portion of the gland secreting glucocorticoids, mineralocorticoids, and sex hormones. The adrenal **medulla** is the inner portion secreting epinephrine and norepineph-rine. (See Appendix F, Figure 7.)

apocrine g.: a type of exocrine gland that loses some of its cellular structure when secreting its product. Examples include sweat glands, ceruminous glands, and mammary glands. **Apo-** means "away from," "derived from."

Bartholin's g.: two small glands located on either side of the vaginal orifice. These glands secrete a fluid that lubricates the vagina, preparing it for intercourse.

bulbourethral g.: an accessory organ of the male repro-ductive system. Secreting a fluid that becomes part of the semen. Also known as *Cowper's gland*. (See Appendix F, Figure 17.)

Cowper's g.: see **bulbourethral gland**

eccrine g.: an exocrine gland that secretes sweat during physical exertion; functions in temperature regulation.

endocrine g.: glands that secrete hormones directly into the blood. Examples include the pituitary, thyroid, parathyroid, thymus, adrenal, pancreas, ovaries, and testes. These hormones have an effect on target cells at some distance from the gland.

exocrine g.: glands that secrete chemicals through ducts onto the surface of the skin or other organ. Examples include sweat, ceruminous, and sebaceous glands.

holocrine g.: a type of exocrine gland in which the secretions contain entire secreting cells. Example, sebaceous glands. **Hol/o** means "whole."

lacrimal g.: glands above the eye that produce tears.

mammary g.: the female breasts that secrete milk.

meibomian g.: glands located in the eyelid that secrete the sebaceous fluid that keeps the lids from sticking to each other. Also known as *tarsal glands*.

merocrine g.: a type of exocrine gland in which the secretion of substances is through the plasma membrane. For example, portions of the pancreas. **Mer/o** means "part."

mixed g.: glands that have both endocrine and exocrine secretions.

parathyroid g.: one of four endocrine glands embedded in the thyroid; secretes parathyroid hormone. (See Appendix F, Figure 7.)

parotid g.: salivary glands located beside the ear. (See Appendix F, Figure 6.)

pineal g.: endocrine gland located in the central portion of the brain secreting melatonin. (See Appendix F, Figure 7.)

Memory Key: The pineal gland is so named because the gland resembles a pine cone.

pituitary g.: an endocrine gland located under the hypothalamus. Also known as the *hypophysis*. (See Appendix F, Figure 7.) The pituitary gland is divided into the ***anterior pituitary*** (adenohypophysis), which produces and secretes numerous hormones (growth hormone, thyrotrophin, adrenocorticotrophic hormone, follicular stimulating hor-

mone, luteinizing hormone, prolactin, and melanocyte stimulating hormone), and the **posterior pituitary** (neurohypophysis), which releases two hormones (oxytocin and
antidiuretic hormone) produced in the hypothalamus and
stored in the posterior pituitary.

prostate g.: male reproductive gland that surrounds the
urethra and the neck of the bladder, secreting fluid that ensures the viability and mobility of sperm. (See Appendix F,
Figure 17.)

salivary g.: three pairs of glands that secrete saliva into the
mouth via ducts. Includes the:

> **parotid g.:** located beside the ear. (See Appendix F,
> Figure 6.) **Para-** means "beside," **ot/o** means "ear."
> **submandibular g.:** located under the lower jaw. (See
> Appendix F, Figure 6.)
> **sublingual g:** located under the tongue. (See Appendix
> F, Figure 6.)

sebaceous g.: exocrine gland that secretes sebum onto
the skin surface through ducts. (See Appendix F, Figure 22.)

sexual g.: ovaries and testicles. Also known as *gonads*.

sudoriferous g.: sweat glands secreting sweat through
pores. Also known as *sweat glands*. (See Appendix F, Figure
22.) Two types of sudoriferous glands are eccrine and apocrine glands.

sweat g.: sudoriferous glands. (See Appendix F, Figure 22.)

tarsal g.: see **gland, meibomian**.

thymus g.: organ located in the mediastinum above the
heart; secretes the hormone thymosin and is the site of
T-lymphocyte production. (See Appendix F, Figure 7.)

thyroid g.: endocrine gland located in the neck below the
larynx and anterior to the trachea; secretes hormones thyroxin, triiodothyronine, and calcitonin. (See Appendix F,
Figure 7.)

glans penis
The tip of the penis. (See Appendix F,
Figure 17.)

glaucoma
A condition of the eye characterized by
increased intraocular pressure resulting in damage to the retina
and optic nerve.

glenoid cavity, glenoid fossa The arm socket; depression on the scapula into which the head of the humerus fits.

gli/o glue
*gli*oma a tumor made up of neuroglial cells
neuro*glia* type of nerve cell. See **neur/o**; **neuroglia**

globulin A plasma protein produced in the liver. Types include alpha, beta, and gamma globulin. Functions include blood clotting, transport, and defense against disease.

glomerul/o glomerulus
*glomerul*ar **capsule** a bowl-shaped structure that surrounds the glomerulus. The filtrate that passes through the walls of the glomerulus falls into the glomerular capsule. Also known as *Bowman's capsule*.
*glomerul*ar **filtration rate (GFR)** the rate in which the filtrate is formed in the glomerulus
*glomerul*onephritis inflammation of the glomeruli
*glomerul*us a cluster of capillaries found in each nephron of the kidney. Functions to start filtration of blood plasma.

Memory Key: -us is a noun ending.

gloss/o tongue
*gloss*ectomy partial or total removal of the tongue
*gloss*itis inflammation of the tongue
*gloss*opharyngeal pertaining to the tongue and pharynx

glottis The slit between the true vocal cords. The glottis opens and closes in the production of speech sounds.

glucagon A hormone produced by the pancreas. Glucagon stimulates the conversion of glycogen to glucose thereby increasing blood glucose.

gluc/o sugar
*gluc*ocorticoids hormones secreted by the adrenal cortex, namely cortisone and cortisol. Necessary for the metabolism

of carbohydrates, fats, and proteins, and for the body's normal response to stress.

glucogenesis production of sugar

gluconeogenesis formation of sugar from fats and proteins

glucose a simple sugar or monosaccharide that is the body's main source of energy. Also known as *dextrose*.

glyc/o sugar

glycolysis breakdown of sugar

glycosuria presence of glucose in the urine

hyper*glycemia* excessive blood sugar

glycogen/o glycogen (storage form of sugar)

glycogenolysis breakdown of glycogen to form glucose

-gnosis knowledge

diagnosis determining the nature of disease. See **dia, diagnosis**.

prognosis prediction or forecast of the outcome of the disease

stereognosis the ability to identify an object by touch alone; visualization of the object is not allowed. **Stere/o** means "solid."

goblet cell A mucus-secreting cell found in the epithelium of the respiratory and intestinal tracts.

goiter Enlarged thyroid gland.

Golgi apparatus An organelle in the cytoplasm of the cell responsible for the secretion of substances out of the cell and the storage of substances within it.

gonad/o gonads

gonadotropin hormones that stimulate the ovaries in the female and the testicles in the male to secrete their own hormones. Includes the follicular stimulating hormone and luteinizing hormone in females and the follicular stimulating hormone and interstitial cell-stimulating hormone in males.

gonads The ovaries and testicles; sexual glands.

goni/o angle of the anterior chamber of the eye between the cornea and iris

gonioscopy process of visually examining the angle of the anterior chamber of the eye with the aid of a gonioscope; a diagnostic examination for glaucoma

gonorrhea A sexually transmitted disease caused by the bacterium *Neisseria gonorrhea.*

gout Dysfunctional metabolism of uric acid that results in abnormal deposits in joint cavities, especially the big toe, causing a form of arthritis.

graafian follicle See **follicle**.

grading of cardiac murmurs An evaluation of the heart's diastolic and systolic murmurs using Arabic numerals. Grades are numbered 1, 2, 3, 4, 5, 6. Grades 1 to 4 for diastolic murmurs (from barely audible to loud). Grades 1 to 6 for systolic murmurs (from barely audible to so loud it can be heard with a stethoscope just above the chest wall).

grading of tumors Evaluating the microscopic appearance of tumor cells to determine the degree of differentiation. Grades are numbered 1, 2, 3, 4. Grades 1 and 2 mean the cells are similar to normal cells and are well differentiated. Grades 3 and 4 mean the cells are abnormal and poorly differentiated compared to normal cells.

graft Tissue that is transplanted into a body part to replace damaged tissue.

-gram record; writing; image

arthrogram x-ray image of a joint following injection of a contrast medium

electrocardiogram (ECG) record of the electrical activity of the heart. See **electr/o, electrocardiogram**.

electroencephalogram (EEG) record of the electrical activity of the brain. See **electr/o, electroencephalogram**.

hysterosalpingogram x-ray image of the uterus and fallopian tubes. See **hyster/o, hysterosalpingogram**.

lymphangiogram x-ray image of the lymph vessels following injection of a contrast medium into a vein

mammogram x-ray image of the breast

myelogram x-ray image of the spinal cord. See **myel/o, myelogram**.

salpingogram x-ray image of the fallopian tube

grand mal seizure   See **seizure**.

-graph instrument used for writing or recording

cardiograph instrument used to record the heart beat

electrocardiograph instrument used to record the electrical activity of the heart

electroencephalograph instrument used to record the electrical activity of the brain

-graphy process of recording; producing images

computed tomography see **tomography**

myelography producing images of the spinal cord by the use of x-rays

mammography producing images of the breast by the use of x-rays

Graves' disease   A disease characterized by overproduction of thyroid hormone, frequently in association with an enlarged thyroid gland (goiter) and protrusion of the eyeballs (exophthalmos).

gravida   A noun meaning the number of times a woman has been pregnant. Written gravida 1, 2 . . . or G1, G2 . . . .

Memory Key: Derived from the Latin *gravis* meaning "heavy or burdensome." Related terms include *grave* (serious), *gravity* (weight).

-gravida number of times a woman has been pregnant

multigravida having been pregnant many times
nulligravida never having been pregnant
primigravida pregnant for the first time
secundigravida pregnant for the second time

gray matter
Material in the brain and spinal cord that is gray in color and consists of unmyelinated fibers and neuron cell bodies.

greater omentum
Peritoneum draping over the intestines. See **omentum**.

greenstick fracture
A partial fracture, which like a green stick or twig from a tree, will bend on one side and break on the other. (See Appendix F, Figure 20.)

growth hormone
Somatotropin. See **somat/o, somatotropin**.

gustatory
Pertaining to the sense of taste.

gynec/o female

gynecologist specialist in the study of diseases and treatment of the female genital tract
gynecology study of diseases and treatment of the female genital tract
gynecomastia abnormal enlargement of the male breast

gyrus
A bulge on the surface of the cerebral cortex. Also known as *a convolution*. (See Appendix F, Figure 11.)

H

hair follicle See **follicle**.

halitosis Bad breath.

hallux great toe
hallux **valgus** see **valgus, hallux valgus**
hallux **varus** see **varum, hallux varus**

hamate One of eight carpal bones. See **carpal bones** under **carp/o**.

haploid A single set of chromosomes. In humans, haploid cells are formed by meiosis and contain 23 chromosomes.

hard palate The bone forming the roof of the mouth.

hare lip A congenital split of the upper lip; cleft lip. See **cheil/o, cheiloschisis**.

haustra Bucketlike pouches that give a distinctive shape to the colon.

Haversian canals A nutrient system of canals within compact bone that contains nerves, blood vessels, and lymphatic vessels.

heart A structure located in the mediastinum that pumps blood through the entire body. (See Appendix F, Figure 4.)

heart block A blockage of electrical impulses anywhere along the conduction system of the heart from the SA node through to the bundle of His.

heartburn See **reflux, gastroesophageal**.

heart failure Failure of the heart to pump sufficient quantities of blood to fill the body's requirement.

heart rate The number of times the heart contracts per minute.

heart sound Two heart sounds created by the closure of the heart valves that are heard through a stethoscope. The first is recognized by a "lupp" sound, the second by a "dubb" sound. The "lupp" sound is the first heart sound (S_1) and represents the closing of the atrioventricular valves; the "dubb" is the second heart sound (S_2) and represents the closing of the semilunar valves.

helper T-lymphocyte Specialized T-lymphocytes that play a role in the cell-mediated immune response by directly destroying virus-infected cells and cancerous cells. Also called *helper T-cells*.

hemi- half

hemianopsia lack of vision in half the visual field

hemicolectomy excision of half the colon

hemiplegia paralysis of either the right or left half of the body

hemisphere half of a spherical organ or structure, such as the right or left cerebral hemispheres

hem/o; hemat/o blood

hemangioma a common benign tumor of blood vessels most often seen in children or infants. Some hemangiomas are known as *nevi*.

hemarthrosis blood in a joint

hematemesis vomiting of blood

hematocele accumulation of blood around the testicles.

hematocrit a laboratory test that determines the percentage of erythrocytes in a blood sample

hematologist one who specializes in the study of the diagnosis and treatment of blood disorders

hematoma accumulation of blood in a space, organ, or tissue due to a break in the blood vessel

Memory Key: Unlike other tumors, a hematoma is not an abnormal growth of tissue but an accumulation of blood into tissues following a ruptured blood vessel. When the word was first used, the bump created by the bleeding into surrounding tissues was thought to be a new growth of cells, hence the use of the suffix **-oma**.

hematopoiesis formation of blood cells

hematosalpinx blood in the fallopian tube

hematuria blood in the urine

hemocytoblast see **stem cells**

hemodialysis (HD) method in which impurities are filtered from the blood by passing it through an artificial kidney machine

hemoglobin a protein found in red blood cells that enables the red blood cell to carry oxygen; pigment in red blood cells that contains iron

hemolysis the breakdown of red blood cells

hemolytic disease of the newborn see **erythroblastosis fetalis** under **erythr/o**

hemopericardium blood in the pericardial sac

hemophilia genetic disorder characterized by the inability of the blood to clot when a vessel is ruptured. Most commonly caused by the lack of clotting factor VIII.

hemoptysis spitting up of blood

hemorrhage bleeding, particularly if it is forceful or severe

hemorrhagic shock see **shock**

hemorrhoid a dilated, varicose vein of the anus

hemostasis to stop the bleeding

hemothorax blood in the pleural cavity

heparin A natural anticoagulant produced by mast cells and basophils. Heparin is also an anticoagulant drug produced by laboratories for therapeutic use.

hepat/o liver

hepatic duct one of the biliary ducts that receives bile from the liver

hepatic flexure bend in the colon under the liver

hepatic portal circulation circulation that reroutes blood from the digestive organs to the liver before returning through veins back to the heart

hepatitis inflammation of the liver

hepatocellular pertaining to liver cells

hepatocyte liver cell

hepatoma tumor of the liver

hepatomegaly enlarged liver

Hering-Breuer reflex A reflex that inhibits
inspiration; therefore, preventing overinflation of the lungs.

herniated disc, herniated nucleus
pulposus A slipped intervertebral disc is characterized
by the herniation or abnormal displacement of the gel-like contents (nucleus pulposusl) of the intervertebral disc through the annulus fibrosus that normally contains it. The displaced nucleus pulposusl pinches the nerve, causing pain.

herni/o hernia

hernia the protrusion or displacement of an organ or part through a structure that normally contains it. Examples include:

diaphragmatic h.: hiatal hernia

hiatal h.: protrusion of abdominal contents into the thorax through the hiatal opening of the diaphragm. Also known as a *diaphragmatic hernia*.

inguinal h.: displacement of abdominal contents into the inguinal canal. Occurs most often in men.

femoral h.: displacement of abdominal contents into the femoral canal of the thigh. Occurs most often in women.

incisional h.: displacement of an organ or part through an incisional site of a previous surgery; ventral hernia

umbilical h.: displacement of abdominal contents through the umbilicus. Most often occurs in newborns.
ventral h.: incisional hernia
herniorrhaphy See **-rrhaphy**

herpes simplex virus (HSV)
A microorganism causing infection of the skin and mucous membrane; HSV, type 1 causes the common cold sore in and around the mouth; HSV, type 2 usually causes herpes genitalis, an infection of the skin and mucous membrane of the genitals; however, some cases of herpes genitalis may be caused by HSV, type 1.

herpes zoster
An infection of the 5th cranial nerve (trigeminal) caused by the varicella-zoster virus, which also causes chicken-pox in children. Also known as *shingles*.

heter/o   another; different
heterogenous of a different species; of different kinds
heterograft surgical graft of tissue between different species

hiatal hernia   See **hernia**.

HIDA scan
A diagnostic imaging technique utilizing a radioactive substance (hepatoiminodiacetic acid) and gamma camera. See **scan**.

high density lipoprotein (HDL)   See **lip/o**; **lipoprotein**.

hilum
A depression in a part of an organ where blood vessels and nerves enter and leave. For example, the hilum of the lung.

hirsutism
Having excessive body or facial hair, particularly in women.

histamine
A natural body substance released by mast cells in response to injury or invasion by foreign substances such as pollen; causes redness, swelling, heat, and pain in body tissues.

histi/o, hist/o tissue

*histi*ocyte a phagocytic cell present in connective tissue
*hist*ology study of tissue

hives See **urticaria**.

Hodgkin's disease Neoplasm of the lymphatic
tissue characterized by enlarged lymph nodes and spleen.

Holter monitor A miniature portable electrocardio-
graphic device that the patient wears for a 24 to 48-hour
period to monitor the action of the heart as the patient goes
through a normal daily routine.

holocrine gland A type of exocrine gland. See
gland.

homeostasis A stable yet varied state of the body.

hom/o same

*homo*genous of the same kind
*homo*logues two members of a chromosome pair
*homo*zygous a condition in which an individual's two alleles
  on a specific gene are identical

hordeolum The inflammation of one or more
sebaceous glands of the eyelid. Also known as a *sty(e)*.

horizontal plane See **plane, transverse**.

hormone A substance produced and secreted by an
endocrine gland, which then travels through the blood to
modify the structure or function of a distant gland or organ.
See specific hormones for definitions.

human immunodeficiency virus (HIV)
A virus that attacks the immune system and causes acquired
immunodeficiency syndrome (AIDS).

human papilloma virus (HPV)   A common
virus causing warts, such as plantar warts, on the sole of the
foot and venereal warts on the penis and female genitalia. See
condyloma acuminatum under **condyl/o**.

humerus   The bone of the upper arm. (See Appendix F,
Figure 19.)

Memory Key: Note the noun ending **-us**. Do not confuse
humerus with the word *humorous* meaning funny.

humoral immunity   See **immunity**.

hyaline   Glasslike cartilage found at the articulating ends of
bones, costal cartilage, larynx, and trachea.

hyaline membrane disease   A respiratory
problem of the premature newborn characterized by collapsed
alveoli due to the lack of surfactant, a substance produced by
the lungs to keep the alveoli inflated. Also known as *respiratory
distress syndrome* (RDS).

hydr/o water

hydrarthrosis accumulation of watery fluid in a joint
hydrocele accumulation of fluid around the testicle.
hydrocephalus accumulation of cerebrospinal fluid in the
brain
hydrochloric acid a substance produced by the stomach,
necessary for the digestion of foods
hydronephrosis accumulation of fluid in the renal pelvis due
to obstruction of the normal urinary pathway
hydrosalpinx watery fluid in the fallopian tube
hydrothorax watery fluid in the pleural cavity

hymen   A layer of mucous membrane that partially or
completely covers the vaginal orifice.

hyoid bone   The horseshoe-shaped bone lying at the
base of the tongue.

hyper- excessive; above; beyond; abnormal increase

hyperbilirubinemia excessive amounts of bilirubin in the blood.

hypercalcemia excessive amounts of calcium in the blood

hypercapnia excessive amounts of carbon dioxide in the blood

hypercholesterolemia excessive amounts of cholesterol in the blood

hyperchromia red blood cells that are darker in color than normal

hyperemesis excessive vomiting

hyperemesis gravidarum excessive vomiting during pregnancy

hyperesthesia increased or exaggerated sensations, particularly a painful sensation from a normally painless touch

hyperextension a joint movement in which the body part is extended beyond its anatomical position

hyperglycemia excessive blood sugar

hyperhidrosis excessive secretion of sweat

hyperkeratosis overgrowth of the stratum corneum. See **kerat/o**.

hyperkinesis abnormally increased muscle activity

hyperlipidemia excessive amount of fats in the blood

hypermetropia farsightedness; an error of refraction in which light rays focus behind the retina making vision of far objects clearer than near objects. Also known as *hyperopia*. Compare with **myopia**.

hyperopia hypermetropia

hyperplasia an abnormal increase in the size of an organ due to an increase in the number of cells, as in malignancy or inflammation. Compare with **hypertrophy**.

hyperpnea abnormal increase in the depth and rate of breathing

hypersensitivity a condition in which the immune system produces tissue damage and disordered function rather than immunity. Also known as an *allergy*.

hypertension high blood pressure; blood pressure greater than 140/90

hypertrophy an abnormal increase in the size of an organ due to an increase in the size of cells. Compare with **hyperplasia**.

Memory Key: Body builders have abnormally large muscles; these muscles are hypertrophied.

hyperventilation abnormally rapid, deep breathing

hyphemia; hyphema Bleeding into the anterior chamber of the eye; blood-shot eyes.

hypo- below; under; deficient; below normal

hypochondriac an individual possessing an abnormal or excessive fear of disease, especially when appearing healthy

Memory Key: In ancient medicine, the spleen was considered to be the site from which melancholy arose. Since the spleen is located in the hypochondrium (abdominal region below the ribs), the term *hypochondriac* was applied.

hypochondrium the upper right and left abdominal areas located below the ribs

hypochromia red blood cells that are lighter in color than normal

hypodermic under the skin

hypoesthesia decreased sensations, particularly to touch

hypogastrium area of the abdomen located below the umbilicus. Compare with **epigastrium** under **epi-**.

Memory Key: In this case **gastr/o** means "belly" referring to the umbilicus.

hypoglycemia deficient amounts of blood sugar

hypokalemia abnormally low concentration of potassium in the blood

hyponatremia abnormally low concentration of sodium in the blood

hypoparathyroidism condition characterized by a deficient secretion of parathormone, resulting in a calcium imbalance

hypophysis pituitary gland

hypospadias congenital opening of the urinary meatus on the ventral (underside) of the penis. Compare with **epispadias** under **epi-**.

hypothalamus portion of the brain located below the thalamus; controls appetite, body temperature, thirst, sleep, and secretions from the pituitary gland. It is also associated with basic behavior patterns.

hypothyroidism condition characterized by deficient secretions of the thyroid hormones: thyroxine and triiodothyronine

hypovolemic shock condition in which a reduction in blood volume leads to a reduction in blood pressure. See **shock**.

hypoxemia deficient amounts of oxygen in the blood

hypoxia lack of or deficiency of oxygen; may be used interchangeably with **anoxia**

hyster/o uterus

hysterectomy surgical removal or excision of the uterus

hysterosalpingectomy surgical removal or excision of the uterus and fallopian tube(s)

hysterosalpingogram record or image produced of the uterus and fallopian tubes by the use of x-rays following injection of a contrast medium through the vagina into the uterus and fallopian tubes

hysterosalpingography process of recording the uterus and tubes following injection of a contrast medium through the vagina

-iasis abnormal condition

candid*iasis* fungal infection caused by *Candida*. See **candid/o**.

cholecystolith*iasis* abnormal condition of stones in the gallbladder; gallstones

iatr/o physician; medical treatment

iatrogenic adverse conditions produced by the patient's contact with physicians or any medical treatment, especially infections passed on by health professionals during treatment or adverse drug reactions

ICSH See **inter-, interstitial-cell stimulating hormone**.

icterus See **jaundice**.

idi/o one's own; of an individual

idiopathic unknown cause; unique to the individual

Memory Key: Related term is *idiosyncrasy* meaning "peculiar to an individual."

ile/o ileum

ileal pertaining to the ileum
ileum third segment of the small intestine. See Memory Key under **ili/o, ilium**.
ileocecal valve valve between the ileum and cecum that functions to keep digested food moving forward
ileostomy creation of a new opening between the ileum and abdominal wall; a type of anastomosis.
ileotomy to cut into the ileum; to incise the ileum
ileus obstruction of the intestine

ili/o hip; ilium

iliac pertaining to the hip
iliofemoral pertaining to the hip and femur
iliosacral joint union between the iliac and sacral bones; sacroiliac joint
ilium one of the bones of the pelvis; the hip bone

Memory Key: Ileum and ilium sound the same but are spelled differently. To remember which means intestine and which word means hip, connect the **e** in il**e**um with the **e** in int**e**stine and the **i** in il**i**um with the **i** in h**i**p.

immune system See **system**.

immunity
Protection against infectious diseases. Types include:

acquired i.: immunity in which the production of antibodies is stimulated following infection by a disease; includes active and passive immunity.

active i.: immunity in which the individual produces his/her own antibodies in response to the disease acquired by natural infection (natural acquired immunity) or vaccination (artificial acquired immunity).

cell-mediated i.: T-lymphocytes are involved in this immune response; antigens are destroyed by direct action on cells.

humoral i.: B-lymphocytes are involved in this immune response; B cells are transformed into plasma cells and secrete antibodies.

natural i.: immunity the individual is born with; does not include antibodies and is genetic in origin.

passive i.: immunity in which the individual acquires antibodies from a donor. For example, in the placental transmission of antibodies from mother to fetus (natural passive immunity) or injection of preformed antibodies after presumed exposure, providing immediate antibody protection (artificial passive immunity).

immun/o immunity; safe

*immun*ization the process of protecting the body against disease

*immuno*deficiency inadequate immune response

*immuno*globulin (Ig) see **gamma globulin**

*immuno*suppressant an agent, such as a drug, used to inhibit the immune system of a patient

impetigo
Superficial but highly contagious skin lesions caused by staphylococcus or streptococcus.

implantation
The process by which the blastocyst (ball of cells formed by the repeated divisions of the fertilized ovum) becomes embedded in the uterine wall.

impotence Male sexual dysfunction characterized by the inability to maintain an erection for intercourse.

in- in; into

*in*cise to cut into; incisors are teeth that can cut into any food for digestion

*in*cisional hernia see **hernia**

*in*semination the placement of sperm into the female reproductive tract by natural or artificial means

in situ confined to the site of origin. For example, carcinoma in situ refers to cancerous cells that have not spread (metastasized) from their original site

*in*spiration to breath air into the lungs; inhalation

in utero in the uterus

*in*version process of turning in; applied to the turning of the sole of the foot inward toward the midline

in vitro occurrence or observation occurring in a test tube (*vitro* means "glass") or other artificial environment; in vitro testing is done in a laboratory setting rather than in the body. For example, at the time of in vitro fertilization (IVF), extracted ova are fertilized by spermatozoa outside the body, usually in a Petri dish. The fertilized ova are then injected into the uterus via the cervix.

in vivo occurrence or observation in a living body (**vivo** means "living body"). For example, in radiology, a contrast study is a diagnostic procedure in which a contrast medium is placed into the patient's body and x-rays are taken of the internal structures. The contrast medium serves to highlight organs that would normally be difficult to visualize.

in- no; not

*in*complete fracture a fracture line that does not involve the whole bone

*in*continence inability to retain urine or feces due to the loss of sphincter control

*in*digestion a vague abdominal discomfort following meals; inability to digest food

*in*fertility the inability to become pregnant

inorganic compound substance that does not contain carbon

irreducible not reducible; not capable of being restored to its normal position, as in an irreducible fracture or hernia

Memory Key: **n** changes to **r** before roots starting with **r**.

incus A tiny bone (ossicle) of the middle ear. Also known as *anvil*. (See Appendix F, Figure 14.)

infarction An area of tissue that has died due to the lack of oxygen supply. An adjective is used to describe the location of the infarction. For example:

cerebral i.: affects the brain

myocardial i.: affects the heart

pulmonary i.: affects the lung

infer/o below

inferior pertaining to below or in a downward position; a structure below another structure

inflammation The body's natural response to injury or infection characterized by redness, swelling, heat, and pain.

Memory Key: infla**mm**ation is spelled with two **m**s; infla**m**ed is spelled with one **m**.

infra- below; beneath

infraclavicular below the clavicle or collarbone

infracostal below the ribs

infraorbital beneath the orbit (eye socket)

infrapatellar below the knee

infraspinous beneath the scapular spine (shoulder blade)

infundibulum The funnel-shaped, distal portion of the fallopian tube.

inguin/o groin

*inguin*al **canal** one-inch long tubular structure on either side of the lower abdominal wall for the passage of the spermatic cord in the male and round ligament in the female

*inguin*al **hernia** see **hernia**

*inguin*al **ring** openings on either side of the inguinal canal

inner cell mass
A mass of cells in the blastocyst from which a new individual develops.

innominate bone
The hip bone; os coxa. (See Appendix F, Figure 19.)

insertion
The point of muscle attachment to the bone that does move. Compare with **origin**.

inspection
The process of examining closely. Inspection is one of four techniques used during the physical examination as an aid to diagnosis. The other techniques include palpation (feel), percussion (tapping), and auscultation (listening). Together with inspection, the entire process can be abbreviated IPPA.

inspiratory reserve volume (IRV)
See **pulmonary function** test under **pulmon/o**.

insular lobe
A lobe embedded deep within the cerebrum; insula.

insulin
A hormone secreted by the pancreas, specifically the beta cells of the islets of Langerhans, to regulate blood glucose levels.

Memory Key: The root **insul/o** means "island." Insulin is so named because it is secreted by the islets (small islands) of Langerhans in the pancreas.

insulin shock
A condition in which an overdose of insulin results in the lowering of blood sugar, which leads to a variety of symptoms, including tachycardia, irritability, tremors, and dizziness. If left untreated, the patient may become comatose.

integumentary system See **system**.

inter- between

interarticular pertaining to between joint surfaces

interatrial septum wall between the atria of the heart

intercalated disc a structure extending between cardiac muscle cells

intercellular between cells

interneuron nerve cell that carries impulses between a sensory and motor neuron

interphalangeal pertaining to between the phalanges

interphase the resting phase in the process of mitosis

interstitial cells cells found in the testicles that produce testosterone. Also known as *Leydig cells* or *interstitial cells of Leydig*.

interstitial-cell stimulating hormone (ICSH) the luteinizing hormone in males secreted by the anterior pituitary. So named because it stimulates the interstitial cells of the testicles to produce testosterone.

interstitial fluid fluid found in the spaces between the cells. This excess fluid filters through the blood capillaries into the lymphatic system becoming lymph.

interventricular septum wall separating the right and left ventricles

intervertebral disc a shock-absorbing fibrocartilaginous disc found between each vertebra; consists of the nucleus pulposus surrounded by the annulus fibrosus

interferon A natural cellular protein formed when cells are exposed to a virus.

interleukin A protein that activates the immune response and stimulates the growth of T-lymphocytes.

internal medicine The branch of medicine dealing with the diagnosis and treatment of diseases of internal structures of the body.

internal respiration See **respiration**.

interoceptor Sensory receptors that receive information about the internal organs; proprioceptor.

intestine That portion of the digestive tract extending from the pyloric sphincter of the stomach to the anus. Includes the small intestine (duodenum, jejunum, ileum) and large intestine (cecum, ascending colon, transverse colon, descending colon, sigmoid colon, rectum, and anus.) Also known as *bowel* or *gut*.

intra- within

intra-**articular** within a joint

intra-**articular fracture** a fracture line that is on the joint surface of the bone

*intra*cellular within the cell

*intra*cranial within the skull

*intra*muscular within a muscle

*intra*ocular within the eyeball

*intra*uterine within the uterus

*intra*uterine device (IUD) a device inserted into the uterus by a physician to help prevent pregnancy

*intra*venous within a vein

intravenous pyelogram (IVP) an x-ray of the urinary tract. See **excretory urogram** under **ur/o**

intravenous urogram (IVU) an x-ray of the urinary tract. See **excretory urogram** under **ur/o**

intrinsic factor A substance secreted by the stomach, necessary for the absorption of vitamin B_{12} in the small intestine.

introitus The entrance to the vagina that is covered by the hymen.

intussusception The telescoping of one portion of the intestine into another.

involuntary muscle A muscle that moves without conscious control, for example, cardiac and visceral muscles.

involution (1) The return of an organ to its normal size after enlargement, particularly the involution of the uterus following delivery of the fetus. (2) The withering of an organ due to old age as in the involuted ovary in postmenopausal women.

iodine See **mineral**.

iodine 131 (^{131}I) A radioisotope used in the diagnosis and treatment of benign and malignant neoplasms of the thyroid gland. See **radioisotope**.

ion An electrically charged atom or molecule.

-ion process
abduction see **abduction** under **ab-**
adduction see **adduction** under **ad-**
agglutination see **agglutination**
alimentation see **alimentation**
retraction see **retraction** under **re-**

ionic bond A type of chemical bond formed between two particles of opposite electrical charge.

IPPA (Inspection, palpation, percussion and auscultation) Four techniques used during the physical examination as an aid to diagnosis. Inspection (to examine), palpation (to feel), percussion (to tap), auscultation (to listen).

irid/o, ir/o iris
iridectomy excision of the iris
iridocyclitis inflammation of the iris and ciliary body
iridotomy incision of the iris
iritis inflammation of the iris

iris The flat circular structure of the eye with a round opening at its center. (See Appendix F, Figure 15.)

iron See **mineral**.

iron deficiency anemia   See **a(n), anemia**.

irradiation   Exposure to radiation.

ischi/o ischium
ischiorectal pertaining to the ischium and rectum
ischium posterior portion of the hip bone. You can feel the
   ischium if you sit on a chair and wriggle your pelvis

isch/o hold back
ischemia inadequate circulation of blood to a part. An adjective is used to describe the location of the ischemia. For
   example:
   myocardial i.: affects the heart
   pulmonary i.: affects the lung
   renal i.: affects the kidney

islets of Langerhans   The cluster of hormone-
producing cells in the pancreas. Includes the alpha cells that
produce and secrete glucagon and beta cells that produce and
secrete insulin.

is/o equal
isometric contraction see **contraction**
isotonic contraction see **contraction**
isotope a chemical element having the same number of pro-
   tons (same atomic number) but a different number of neutrons (different atomic mass) than some other element

isthmus   A narrow, necklike passage connecting two
spaces or cavities. The thyroid isthmus is the central segment of
the gland connecting the right and left lobes.

-itis inflammation
Memory Key: There are hundreds of medical words ending
in **-itis**, too many to list here; however, **-itis** preceded by almost any number of anatomical roots means the inflammation
of that anatomical structure.

aden*itis* inflammation of a gland
appendic*itis* inflammation of the appendix
cyst*itis* inflammation of the bladder
nephr*itis* inflammation of the kidney

IVP intravenous pyelogram See **excretory urogram** under **ur/o**.

IVU intravenous urogram See **excretory urogram** under **ur/o**.

J

jaundice A yellow or orange discoloration of the skin due to high levels of bilirubin in the blood, often resulting from liver disease. Also known as *icterus*.

jejunu/o jejunum

jejunum the second of three segments of the small intestine. (See Appendix F, Figure 6.)

Memory Key: Note the noun ending **-um**.

joint The juncture between two bones; an articulation.

juxtaglomerular apparatus A collection of cells surrounding the arteriole leading to the glomerulus of the kidney, consisting of specialized cells that secrete renin and aid in controlling the glomerular filtration rate.

K

Kaposi's sarcoma A malignant tumor arising from the lining of capillaries, characterized by purple discoloration of skin; most commonly seen as an opportunistic disease found in AIDS patients.

kary/o nucleus

karyocyte a nucleated cell

karyoplasm protoplasm found in the nucleus of the cell; nucleoplasm

karyotype the full chromosome set of a given individual

keloid scar An abnormally large and thick scar development of the skin due to overactive collagen formation during tissue repair following injury.

kerat/o, keratin/o hard; hornlike

hyper*kerat*osis overgrowth of the stratum corneum, the outermost, hornlike layer of the epidermis

keratin a protein found in the epidermis and nails that makes them tough, waterproof, and resistant to bacteria

Memory Key: Do not confuse **keratin** with the similar-sounding word **carotene**, which is a yellow pigment in tissues.

keratinocytes cells in the epidermis that produce keratin

keratolysis destruction or separation of the outermost, horn-like layer of the epidermis

keratosis thickening of the epidermis as in warts or calluses

kerat/o cornea

keratoconjunctivitis inflammation of the cornea and conjunctiva

keratoconus a cone-shaped protrusion in the center of the cornea

keratomycosis fungal infection of the cornea

*kerato*plasty procedure involving the replacement of a dysfunctional, nontransparent cornea with a normal, transparent cornea in an effort to restore vision; also called *corneal transplant*

ket/o

ketoacidosis accumulation of ketones in the body leading to coma and death; a complication of advanced diabetes mellitus

ketones
End product of fat metabolism sometimes referred to as acetones.

kidney
Bean-shaped, fist-sized structures lying on each side of the lumbar vertebra. Functions to form urine and filter out waste products from the blood. (See Appendix F, Figure 23.)

killer T-lymphocytes
A blood cell important in the cell-mediated immune response. It kills some cancerous cells and cells that have been infected by fungi, parasites, or viruses. Also called *cytotoxic T-lymphocyte*.

kilocalorie
(1) Used to express the fuel or energy value of food. Also known as *calorie*. (2) The amount of heat required to raise the temperature of one kilogram of water one degree Celsius.

kilogram
1000 grams or approximately 2.2 pounds.

kinesi/o movement

a**kinesia** lack of movement
dys**kinesia** impaired muscle movement
kinesiology study of muscles and muscular movement
kinesiometer instrument used to measure movement

knee jerk
See **reflex, patellar**.

knock-kneed
See **genu, genu valgum**.

Krebs cycle A series of reactions in the mitochondria resulting in the liberation of energy to be used by the body. Also known as the *citric acid cycle* or *tricarboxylic acid cycle*.

Kupffer's cell Phagocytic liver cells that detoxify harmful substances.

kyphosis Exaggerated posterior curvature of the thoracic spine; humpback.

L

labi/o lips
*labi*al pertaining to a lip
labia **majora** larger, outermost lips of the external female genitalia
labia **minora** smaller, innermost lips of the external female genitalia
*labi*oglossopharyngeal pertaining to the lips, tongue, and throat

labor The process by which the fetus is expelled from the uterus and vagina to the outside of the body; the birth process. Also known as *parturition*.

labyrinth The inner ear, consisting of a system of passageways or canals; includes the **membranous labyrinth** surrounded by the **bony labyrinth**. Functions to maintain balance. (See Appendix F, Figure 14.)

labyrinth/o inner ear; labyrinth
*labyrinth*itis inflammation of the inner ear

labyrinthotomy incision into the inner ear

laceration A wound with jagged edges.

lacrim/o tears

lacrimal **apparatus** structures that produce, secrete, and transport tears. Includes the lacrimal glands, lacrimal ducts, punctae, lacrimal canals, lacrimal sac, and nasolacrimal duct.

lacrimal **canal** passageway for tears leading from the eye to the nose

lacrimal **duct** passageway for tears leading from the lacrimal gland to the eye

lacrimal **gland** gland above the eye that produces tears

lacrimal **sac** bulbous, proximal portion of the nasolacrimal duct

naso*lacrimal* duct duct that drains tears from the lacrimal sac into the nasal cavity

lact/o milk

lactase an enzyme that converts glucose to galactose

lactation period during which milk is secreted; milk secretion

lacteal lymphatic vessel that carries chyle (intestinal lymph) from the intestines

Memory Key: The presence of fat gives chyle a milky appearance, hence the name *lacteal*.

lactiferous **duct** tube that carries milk from the lobes of the breast to the nipple

lactogenesis production of milk

lactose a disaccharide found in milk

pro*lactin* hormone produced by the anterior pituitary

lacuna A small hollow space. In bone, the lacunae are spaces in the bony matrix that contain an osteocyte.

Laënnec's cirrhosis Chronic degeneration of the liver due to alcoholism.

lambdoidal suture The immovable joint of the skull. See **suture**, definition (3).

lamella A thin concentric circle of osseous tissue surrounding the Haversian canal.

lamina propria The thin layer of fibrous connective tissue that underlies the surface epithelium of mucous membranes.

lapar/o abdomen

laparoscope an instrument similar to a telescope that is inserted into the abdomen through a small incision in the abdominal wall. It is equipped with a light and a cutting instrument to allow destruction or removal of tissue without opening up the abdominal cavity.

laparoscopy process of viewing the abdominal cavity by inserting a laparoscope through a small abdominal incision near the umbilicus. This procedure may be performed for diagnosis of disease, for tubal ligation, for the removal of body tissues or organs such as the gallbladder, or for destruction of tissue using laser.

laparotomy incision into the abdominal wall

laryng/o larynx; voicebox

laryngitis inflammation of the larynx

laryngopharynx lower portion of the pharynx

laryngospasm sudden, violent, muscular contractions of the larynx blocking air flow

laryngotracheobronchitis a condition in which inflammation of the larynx, trachea, and bronchus obstruct the upper respiratory tract. Commonly seen in infants and young children. Also known as *croup*.

larynx The part of the respiratory tract that connects the pharynx with the trachea. (See Appendix F, Figure 18.)

laser An instrument used for cutting, hemostasis, and destruction of tissue with light rays. Laser is an acronym that has been accepted as a word. It is short for light amplification by stimulated emission of radiation.

laser **iridectomy** use of a laser to surgically remove a portion of the iris.

laser **photocoagulation** procedure in which a laser is used to coagulate tissue in the interior of the eye. Used to treat retinal tears.

later/o side

lateral pertaining to the side; a directional term referring to a position away from the midline of the body or organ

lateral **horn** gray matter in the spinal cord between the anterior and posterior horns

lavage
To irrigate or wash out an organ, such as the stomach. See **gastric lavage** under **gastr/o**.

lei/o smooth muscle

leiomyoma benign tumor of smooth muscle. Frequently occurs in the uterus. Also known as *fibroids, uterine myomas, leiomyoma uteri,* or *fibromyomas.*

leiomyosarcoma malignant tumor of smooth muscle

lens
The transparent structure of the eye located posterior to the pupil and iris. The lens refracts light rays and changes its shape (accommodation) in order to focus a sharp image on the retina, whether the objects are near or far. (See Appendix F, Figure 15.)

lesion
Any deviation from the normal appearance of the skin; can be congenital or caused by disease or injury. Examples include macules, papules, and pustules.

lesser omentum
The peritoneal membrane in the abdominal cavity. See **omentum**.

leuk/o white

leukemia a malignant increase in the number of white blood cells; considered a cancer

leukoblast immature white blood cell

leukocyte mature white blood cell

leukocytopenia deficiency in the number of white blood cells; leukopenia

leukocytosis slight increase in the number of white blood cells caused by such conditions as fever, hemorrhage, infection, and inflammation. The use of the word *slight* is relative as leukocytosis is a slight increase as compared to leukemia, which is a malignant increase of white blood cells.

leukoderma lack of pigmentation in the skin showing up as white patches. Also known as *vitiligo*.

leukopenia leukocytopenia

leukoplakia white patches on mucous membrane. **-plakia** means "patches."

leukopoiesis production of leukocytes

leukorrhea whitish flow or discharge from the vagina

Leydig cells
Testicular cells that secrete testosterone; interstitial cells of Leydig.

ligament
A fibrous band of connective tissue connecting bone to bone.

ligament/o
ligamentoplasty surgical reconstruction of a ligament

limbic system
A structure deep in the cerebrum near the brain stem. The limbic system includes the basal ganglia, thalamus, hypothalamus, amygdala, fornix, cingulate gyrus, and hippocampus; involved in the control of emotions and autonomic functions.

linea line
linea alba vertical, white line of connective tissue in the middle of the abdomen from the sternum to the pubis. The linea alba is formed by the intertwining of muscle fibers from the right and left abdominal sides.

linea aspera a rough edge located on the posterior surface of the middle third of the femur

linear fracture A fracture in which the fracture line runs parallel to the axis of the bone.

lingu/o tongue

lingual **tonsils** mass of lymphatic tissue on the base of the tongue

sub*lingual* pertaining to under the tongue

lip (1) The soft external folds around the mouth. (2) The lips of external female genitalia.

lip/o fat

lipase enzyme that changes fats into fatty acids and glycerol

lipid fatty compound

lipoma a benign tumor composed of fat cells. Also known as *steatoma*.

lipoprotein fat and protein complex transported through the blood

high density l. (HDL): removes excess cholesterol from the walls of an artery and transports it to the liver, thereby protecting the adult from atherosclerosis.

low density l. (LDL) and **very low density l. (VLDL):** both these lipoproteins are linked to atherosclerosis.

liposuction withdrawal of fat from subcutaneous tissue. Liposuction is considered a cosmetic surgery to enhance body shape and contour.

lith/o stone; calculus

lithiasis condition of stones in the kidney or gallbladder

lithotomy incision into an organ, especially the bladder, for the removal of stones

lithotomy **position** a surgical position in which the patient lies face upward with thighs flexed onto the abdomen and abducted. Most often used in gynecological procedures.

lithotripsy the crushing of kidney stones or gallstones

percutaneous ultrasonic l.: crushing of kidney stones or gallstones using ultrasound that travels through the skin and onto the stones.

liver The largest solid organ in the body, located in the right upper quadrant of the abdomen.

lob/o lobe

lobar **pneumonia** inflammation of one or more lobes of the lung

lobe A small section of an organ.

lobectomy partial or complete surgical removal of a lobe of the lung

lobes **of cerebrum** the cerebrum is divided into lobes generally named after the bony structures that lie above. Included are the

    frontal l.: front of the cerebrum, functions in voluntary movements and speech movements.

    insular l.: embedded deep in the cerebrum

    parietal l.: posterior to frontal lobe, functions in skin sensations, and muscle awareness.

    occipital l.: at the back of the cerebrum functions in vision.

    temporal l.: at the sides of the cerebrum, functions in hearing, smell, and taste.

lobule a small lobe as seen in the liver

local Confined to a specific body region or organ.

loins Area of the back between the ribs and hip.

loop of Henle The u-shaped, ascending and descending limbs of the nephron.

lordosis Exaggerated anterior curvature of the lumbar spine; swayback.

low density lipoprotein (LDL) See **lip/o, lipoproteins**.

lower esophageal sphincter The circular muscle at the distal esophagus. See **sphincter, cardiac**.

lumb/o lower back; loin

lumbago pain in the loins; lumbodynia

lumbar pertaining to the loins, the area of the back between the ribs and hip

lumbar plexus network of nerves in the lower back. See **plexus**.

lumbar puncture (LP) insertion of a needle into the subarachnoid space below L3 to withdraw cerebrospinal fluid for diagnostic or therapeutic purposes. Also called a *spinal tap*.

lumbar vertebrae five spinal bones of the lower back. See **vertebra**. (See Appendix F, Figure 21.)

lumbodynia lumbago

lumen
The area within a tube through which substances pass, such as within a vein, artery, or intestine.

lunate
One of eight carpal bones. See **carpal bones** under **carp/o**.

lung
An organ of respiration located in the thoracic cavity. The right and left lung are separated by the mediastinum. (See Appendix F, Figure 18.)

lunula
The half-moon shaped white area at the base of the finger- or toenail.

luteinizing hormone
A gonadotrophic hormone produced by the anterior pituitary gland that promotes ovulation in females and stimulates hormonal secretion by the testicles in males. In males, the luteinizing hormone is also called *interstitial cell-stimulating hormone* (ICSH).

lymph
A clear colorless fluid in the lymph vessels; it is similar to plasma but lacks plasma proteins.

lymphaden/o lymph nodes
lymphadenitis inflammation of the lymph nodes

lymphadenopathy any disease of the lymph nodes, particularly enlargement of the lymph nodes

lymphangi/o lymph vessels

lymphangiography x-ray of the lymph vessels and lymph
nodes following injection of a contrast medium into the feet.
The contrast medium moves upward through the lymphatic
system into all areas of the body.

lymphangiitis; lymphangitis inflammation of the lymph
vessels

lymphatic ducts

left lymphatic duct: drains lymph from the entire body
except the right head and neck, right arm, and right chest.
Also known as the *thoracic duct*. (See Appendix F, Figure 8.)

right lymphatic duct: drains lymph from the right
head and neck, right arm, and right chest. (See Appendix F,
Figure 8.)

lymphatic system See **system**.

lymph nodes Oval-shaped structures that remove
unwanted substances, such as bacteria and toxins, from lymph.
Located in clusters, lymph nodes are named according to their
location, such as cervical, submandibular, axillary, and inguinal
lymph nodes. (See Appendix F, Figure 8.)

lymph/o

lymphangiogram record of the lymph vessels following
injection of a contrast medium into a vein

lymphedema accumulation of fluid due to obstruction of
lymphatic structures

lymphoblast immature lymphocyte (white blood cell)

lymphocyte a nongranular leukocyte; a type of white blood
cell

lymphocytopenia lymphopenia

lymphokine chemical produced by T-cell lymphocytes in cell-
mediated immunity that has a destructive effect on antigens

lymphoma malignant tumor of the lymph nodes and lymph
tissue

lymphopenia deficiency of lymphocytes in the blood;
lymphocytopenia

lymph vessels A series of tubes that collects lymph in tissues and transports them into veins of the cardiovascular system. Lymph vessels include lymph capillaries, lymphatics, and lymphatic ducts. (See Appendix F, Figure 8.)

-lysis breakdown; separation

acantholysis breakdown of the prickle-cell layer of the skin

dialysis mechanical replacement of kidney function when the kidney is dysfunctional; literally, **dialysis** means "to separate apart"

hemolysis breakdown of blood

glycogenolysis breakdown of glycogen to form glucose

lipolysis breakdown of fat

rhabdomyolysis breakdown of striated muscle tissue

urinalysis analysis of urine

lys/o dissolution; breakdown

lysosome organelle of the cytoplasm containing enzymes that destroy bacteria, viruses, and worn-out organelles. Sometimes called *suicide bags* or *garbage bags*.

lysozyme an enzyme in tears and saliva that damages bacterial cells

macro- large

macrocephalia excessively large head for the rest of the body

macrophage large phagocytes that destroy worn-out red blood cells and engulf foreign material in body tissues

macroscopic large enough to be seen with the unaided eye

macula densa A group of closely packed cells in the wall of the distal convoluted tubule of the nephron. Associated with the juxtaglomerular apparatus, the **macula densa**

contributes to the kidney's endocrine function and controls the glomerular filtration rate.

macula lutea The small, yellowish area near the center of the retina containing the fovea centralis, in which a high number of cones are located allowing for sharp and focused vision.

macular degeneration The degradation of the retinal cells in the macula lutea of the eye that results in a loss of central vision.

macule Skin lesion characterized by a discolored, unelevated area of skin. Example, birthmarks. A lesion greater than 1 cm is called a "patch."

magnesium See **mineral**.

magnetic resonance imaging (MRI) A noninvasive diagnostic procedure using radiofrequency waves and a strong magnetic field to produce clear images of body structures, particularly the brain, heart, blood vessels, and soft tissue.

-malacia softening

cerebromalacia softening of brain tissue, particularly the cerebrum
chondromalacia softening of cartilage
osteomalacia softening of bone
phacomalacia softening of the lens of the eye

malaise A general feeling of bodily discomfort ; literally means "ill at ease."

Memory Key: Common English words using **mal-** are **mal**ice (ill-will) and **mal**ady (an illness).

malignant The tendency to grow worse; said of cancerous tumors, which have the malignant characteristics of anaplasia (undifferentiated cells) and metastasis (spreading to other sites). Compare with **benign**.

malleolus A rounded process on either side of the ankle joint; includes the medial and lateral malleolus.

malleus The tiny bone (ossicle) of the middle ear. Also known as the *hammer*. (See Appendix F, Figure 14.)

maltase The enzyme that converts maltose to glucose.

maltose A disaccharide found in malt products; used as a sweetener.

mamm/o, mast/o breast

mammary gland see **gland**
mammogram record of the breast produced using x-rays
mammography process of producing an image of the breast using x-rays
mammoplasty surgical reconstruction of the breast; surgical reduction or augmentation (enlargement) of the breast
mastectomy excision of the breast
mastitis inflammation of the breast

mandibl/o mandible; lower jaw

mandibular pertaining to the lower jaw. Compare with **maxilla**. (See Appendix F, Figure 19.)

mast cells A connective-tissue cell that secretes histamine and heparin.

masticate To chew.

mastoid/o mastoid process

mastoid resembling a breast
mastoiditis inflammation of the air cells of the mastoid process
mastoid process nipple-shaped, rounded process of the temporal bone extending downward behind the ear

matrix A basic substance from which anything is formed or shaped; the intercellular material in a tissue. For example, the bony matrix.

matter Anything that occupies space and has weight.

maxill/o maxilla; upper jaw

maxillary pertaining to the upper jaw. Compare with
  mandible. (See Appendix F, Figure 19.)

Memory Key: To remember that **maxilla** means "upper jaw,"
think of *maximum* meaning "greatest," "highest," or "uppermost."

McBurney's point The area of the abdomen in the
right lower quadrant above the appendix.

meatus An opening or passage. Examples include:

  external auditory m.: bilateral tubes that transmit sound
  waves from the external to the middle ear. (See Appendix F,
  Figure 14.)

  urinary m.: exterior opening of the urethra; in the male it
  is on the tip of the penis, in the female it is anterior to the
  vagina. Also known as *urethral orifice*. (See Appendix F,
  Figure 23.)

mechanoreceptor A neural receptor that
responds to mechanical stimulation such as light and sound.

medi/o middle

medial pertaining to the middle; a directional term referring
  to a position toward the midline of the body or organ

mediastinum; mediastinal cavity The
body cavity between the two lungs containing the heart,
esophagus, trachea, and some large blood vessels.

medulla The inner region of an organ such as the
adrenal medulla and renal medulla.

medulla oblongata The part of the brain stem
just above the spinal cord that serves as a vital link for eyes,
ears, circulatory, respiratory, and skeletal functions. Medullary
fibers carrying electrical impulses cross one side to the other in

the medulla oblongata, and thus the right hemisphere of the brain controls the left side of the body and vice versa. *Oblongata* means "rather long." (See Appendix F, Figure 11.)

medullary cavity The hollow space in the shaft of a long bone containing bone marrow.

megal/o abnormal enlargement

megaloblast immature abnormal red blood cell with a large-sized nucleus

megalocyte abnormally large red blood cell

-megaly abnormal enlargement

acromegaly enlargement of the extremities caused by hyper-secretion of the growth hormone from the pituitary gland; occurs after bones have stopped growing

cardiomegaly enlarged heart

hepatomegaly enlarged liver

splenomegaly enlarged spleen

visceromegaly enlarged internal organs; *organomegaly*

meibomian glands Glands in the eyelid. See **gland**.

meiosis A type of division of sex cells in which there is a reduction in the number of chromosomes by half. When the sperm fertilizes the egg and the zygote is formed, there will be a full chromosome complement.

Meissner's plexus The nerves in the small intestine. See **plexus**.

melan/o black

melanemesis black vomit; dark-colored vomit due to the mixture of vomit with blood

melanin a black pigment that gives color to our skin and hair. Melanin is produced by the melanocytes in the epidermis.

Memory Key: **-in** is a noun suffix for a chemical compound.

melanocytes cells in the epidermis that produce melanin

melanocyte-stimulating hormone hormone produced by the anterior pituitary gland regulating skin pigmentation

melanoma malignant tumor of the skin arising from the melanocytes, chiefly due to overexposure to sunlight

melatonin
A hormone secreted by the pineal gland. In humans it is implicated in seasonal mood changes and sleep.

melena
(1) Black, tarry stools due to the mixing of blood with intestinal juices; feces mixed with blood. (2) Black vomit due to the mixture of blood with gastric contents.

membrane
A thin layer of tissue that covers a structure, lines a cavity, or separates one part from another.

membrane potential
An electrical potential that exists across a cell membrane.

membranous labyrinth
The membranous portion of the inner ear. See **labyrinth**.

memory cell
T and B lymphocytes that play a role in the immune response by retaining information that allows them to combat a disease that has occurred previously in the body.

Ménière's disease
A condition of the inner ear that includes vertigo (dizziness), tinnitus (ringing in the ears), and hearing loss.

meninges
Singular is meninx. Three membranes that protect the brain and spinal cord. (See Appendix F, Figure 12.) Includes:

meningi/o, mening/o meninges; membrane
arachnoid: the middle layer of the meninges

Memory Key: Arachnoid means "resembling a spider." On examination of the arachnoid membrane, anatomists found this layer to resemble a spider web, hence its name.

dura mater: the outermost and toughest of the three meninges that protect the brain and spinal cord. Also known as *pachymeninges*.

Memory Key: Dura mater literally means "tough mother," in the sense of all-protecting mother (of the brain).

pia mater: the thin, delicate innermost membrane covering the brain and spinal cord

Memory Key: Pia mater literally means "tender mother." This relates to the delicate appearance of this membrane.

meningioma a slow-growing, benign tumor of the meninges
meningitis inflammation of the meninges. May be fatal.
meningocele hernia or protrusion of the meninges through an opening in the skull or spinal column
meningoencephalitis inflammation of the meninges and brain
meningomyelocele hernia or protrusion of the meninges and spinal cord through a defect in the skull or vertebral column. Also known as *myelomeningocele*.

meniscus The c-shaped cartilage located at the knee joint between the femur and tibia. Also known as *semilunar cartilage*. Plural is menisci.

men/o month

amenorrhea no menstruation
dysmenorrhea painful menstruation
menarche beginning of the regular menstrual cycle starting approximately at the age of 12
menometrorrhagia irregular and excessive menstrual bleeding
menopause the permanent cessation of menstruation, usually between 50 and 55 years of age
menorrhagia excessive uterine bleeding during menstruation
menorrhea normal menstruation

menstruation periodic shedding of the endometrial lining from the uterus if the ovum is not fertilized

oligomenorrhea scanty uterine bleeding during menstruation

merocrine gland A type of exocrine gland. See **gland**.

mesentery Peritoneum that attaches the small intestine to the posterior abdominal wall, keeping it in position.

meso- middle

mesocolon peritoneum that attaches the colon to the posterior abdominal wall, keeping it in position

mesoderm middle layer of embryonic cells. See **-derm**.

mesoenchyma embryonic tissue in the mesoderm from which all connective tissue arises

mesothelium type of epithelial tissue. See **thel/o**.

meta- beyond; change

metabolism chemical and physical changes occurring in the body

metacarpal bones of the hand. Literally means "beyond the carpal bones." (see Appendix F, Figure 19.)

metacarpophalangeal joint (MCP) junction between the metacarpals and the fingers

metaphase phase two in the process of mitosis, in which the pairs of chromatids line up on the equator of the cell

metaplasia changing of tissue from one form to another form that is not normal for that tissue

metastasis the spread of a malignant tumor from one part of the body to another. Metastasize is the verb.

metatarsal bones of the foot. (See Appendix F, Figure 19.)

Memory Key: **Metatarsal** literally means "beyond the tarsal bones."

metr/o uterus

endometrium inner lining of the uterus

metroptosis drooping of the uterus; uterine prolapse

metrorrhagia irregular uterine bleeding at any time other than during the regular menstrual period

myometrium muscular wall of the uterus

parametrium connective tissue extending from the uterus

perimetrium the outermost wall of the uterus

-metry measure

craniometry process of measuring the skull bones

pelvimetry measurement of the pelvis to confirm the size of the maternal pelvis in situations in which the pelvis is thought to be too small for the delivery of the baby

symmetry see **sym-**

micro- small

microbe a microscopic microorganism

microglia a type of neuroglial cell that is supportive and connective in function. Does not transmit impulses.

microgram (mcg) one-millionth part of a gram. One-thousandth of a milligram.

microscope instrument used to magnify minute objects

microtubule hollow, tubular structure present in a cell important in maintaining cell structure and in converting chemical energy into work

microvilli microscopic, fingerlike projections from the free surface of a cell membrane

micturition Urination.

mid- middle

midbrain middle segment of the brain stem responsible for visual and auditory reflexes, such as moving the head and eyes to view objects or turning of the head so that sound can be heard directly. (See Appendix F, Figure 11.)

midsagittal plane see **plane**.

milli- thousand

milligram (mg) one-thousandth of a gram

milliliter (ml) one-thousandth of a liter

millimeter **(mm)** one-thousandth of a meter

millimol **(mM)** one-thousandth of a mol.

mineral An inorganic solid substance found in nature.
Examples include:

calcium: important in muscle contraction and electrical impulses

chloride: a salt of hydrochloric acid

iodine: important in the production of thyroid hormones, which regulate the metabolic rate in cells

iron: essential to hemoglobin formation and cellular respiration

magnesium: activates enzymes, associated with body temperature, neuromuscular contraction, and protein synthesis

phosphorus: found in almost all tissues, especially bone

Memory Key: Do not confuse phosphor**us**, the noun with phosphor**ous**, the adjective.

potassium: chief alkaline chemical element in intracellular fluid, particularly in muscle; is important in the conduction of nerve impulses.

sodium: chief alkaline chemical element of the extracellular body fluid; is important in initiating an action potential.

zinc: important in protein synthesis and cell division; is an essential element in many enzymes.

mineralocorticoids A classification of hormones
secreted by the adrenal cortex. The most important of these is aldosterone, which regulates the retention and secretion of sodium and potassium.

mi/o contraction; less

miosis abnormal contraction of the pupil

miotic drug used to constrict the pupil

miscarriage Spontaneous abortion; naturally occurring
abortion.

mitochondrion A cytoplasmic organelle that produces most of a cell's ATP, thereby providing energy for the cell through the reactions of the Krebs cycle.

mitosis A type of cell division in which one cell with the diploid number of chromosomes (46 for humans) divides to form two identical cells, each with the diploid number of chromosomes.

mitral valve The valve located between the left atrium and ventricle; bicuspid valve; left atrioventricular valve. (See Appendix F, Figure 4.)

mitral valve incompetence See **mitral valve insufficiency**.

mitral valve insufficiency The inability of the mitral valve to close tightly, resulting in a backflow of blood. Also known as *mitral valve incompetence*.

mitral valve regurgitation The backflow of blood from the left ventricle into the left atrium because of mitral valve insufficiency.

mitral valve stenosis Narrowing of the mitral valve preventing flow of blood through the heart.

mittelschmerz Abdominal pain at time of ovulation.

mixed gland See **gland**.

mixed nerve Nerves that have both sensory (afferent) and motor (efferent) fibers.

molar Teeth used for grinding of food. Molars have three projections or cusps and are also known as *tricuspids*.

mole (1) The mass in grams of an element or compound numerically equivalent to the atomic weight (for elements) or the molecular weight (for compounds.) (2) A pigmented, elevated lesion on the surface of the skin. Also known as a *nevus*.

molecule   Two or more atoms that form a specific chemical compound.

moniliasis   A fungal infection. See **candidiasis**.

mono- one

monoblast   immature monocyte

monocyte   a leukocyte that engulfs bacteria. Formed in the bone marrow, it develops into macrophages in the lung and liver.

monokine   substance produced by monocytes or macrophages to play a role in the immune system by allowing communication between cells

monoplegia   paralysis of one limb

monosaccharide   a simple sugar, one that cannot be decomposed by hydrolysis. Examples are fructose and galactose.

mons pubis   A fatty prominence covered with pubic hair above the symphysis pubis in the female; part of the female external genitalia.

morphology   The study of shape or form.

postmortem; post mortem   After death.

morula   A solid mass of cells in the early stage of embryonic development.

motor neuron   An efferent neuron. See **neuron**.

motor system   An efferent system. See **system**.

motor tract   A bundle of nerve fibers that transmits impulses away from the brain and spinal cord to a muscle.

motor unit A motor neuron plus the muscle fibers it controls.

mouth The oral cavity. (See Appendix F, Figure 6.)

MRI See **magnetic resonance imaging**.

muc/o mucus

*muc*oid resembling mucus
*muc*olytic an agent that breaks down mucus
*muc*osa mucous membrane
*muc*ous adjective form of mucus. See Memory Key below.
*muc*ous membrane membrane that lines cavities leading to
  the exterior, such as the digestive and respiratory tracts.
  Contains cells that secrete mucus. Also known as *mucosa*.

Memory Key: Note the difference in spelling between
muc**us**, the noun, and muc**ous**, the adjective. Spelling errors
are common between these two words, but it is helpful to
remember that **-ous** is the adjectival ending meaning "pertaining to."

*muc*us a thick, slimy secretion from the cells of the mucous
  membrane. Phlegm and secretions from the nose are examples of mucus. See Memory Key under **mucous
  membrane** above.

multi- many

*multi*cellular having many cells
*multi*form having many shapes or forms
*multi*gravida having been pregnant many times
*multi*para having given birth two or more times. See **-para,
  multipara**.
*multi*polar neuron a neuron consisting of many processes
  (axons and dendrites) extending from its cell body

multiple sclerosis A chronic disease characterized
by inflammation of the myelin sheath leading to demyelination
around the axon causing a variety of neurological disorders,
such as visual disturbances, urinary dysfunction, muscle

weakness, and emotional instability. Called **multiple** because there are relapses and remissions of the disease occurring over a long period of time.

murmur   A soft blowing sound; an abnormal heart sound.

muscle   Organs that cause movement by contraction or shortening. Types include:

cardiac m.: found in the heart. Also known as *striated involuntary muscle*. The striated or striped appearance is due to a pattern of dark and light bands; it is under unconscious (involuntary) nervous control.

skeletal m.: muscle lying on top of bone, pulling on bones for movement. Dark and light bands give the muscle a striated or striped appearance; is considered voluntary muscle because it is under conscious nervous control. Also known as *striated voluntary muscle*.

visceral m.: located in internal body organs, such as the stomach, intestines, and blood vessels. Also known as *smooth* or *nonstriated involuntary muscle*. Visceral muscles have a smooth appearance as there are no dark or light bands in the muscle tissue; is considered involuntary muscle because it is under unconscious nervous control.

muscle fatigue   The inability of the muscle fibers to contract due to the lack of oxygen and accumulation of lactic acid.

muscle fiber   A muscle cell. Muscles cells are not spherical, but long and slender; therefore, are often referred to as fibers.

muscle spasm   A sudden, violent, involuntary contraction (shortening) of a muscle.

muscle spindle   A sensory receptor between skeletal muscle fibers.

muscle tissue   Tissue specialized for contraction—causing movement of body parts.

muscle tone The normal flexibility and firmness of muscles; normal low-level tension present in healthy muscle tissues due to their continual and partial contraction.

muscle twitch A brief response of a skeletal muscle to a single stimulus.

muscular system See **system**.

muscul/o muscle

muscular **dystrophy** a genetic disease, most often seen in boys, characterized by the replacement of muscle tissue by fat and fibrous tissue with progressive muscle dysfunction. The skeletal muscles are first affected, followed by the involuntary muscles. In the late stages of the disease, the involuntary muscles of the heart are affected, resulting in eventual heart failure. Most common type is Duchenne's muscular dystrophy.

*musculo*skeletal pertaining to the muscles and skeleton

mutation A change in the DNA; a genetic change that may be passed to offspring.

myc/o fungus

dermato**mycosis** fungal infection of the skin
kerato**mycosis** fungal infection of the cornea
*myc*osis any disease caused by a fungal infection

mydri/o wide; dilatation

*mydri*asis abnormal dilatation of the pupil
*mydri*atic pertaining to a drug used to dilate the pupil

myelin sheath A fatty covering around the axon of some neurons. (See Appendix F, Figure 13.)

myel/o spinal cord; bone marrow

Memory Key: Look at the context of the word in the sentence to decide whether **myel/o** means "spinal cord" or "bone marrow."

demyelination lack of or destruction of the myelin sheath around a nerve fiber. Characteristic of multiple sclerosis.

myeloblast immature bone marrow cell

myelogenous produced by the bone marrow

myelogram record of the spinal cord made by x-rays following injection of a contrast medium into the subarachnoid space at the lumbar area of the back

myelography process of recording images of the spinal cord following injection of contrast medium into the subarachnoid space at the lumbar area of the back

myeloma tumor composed of cells normally found in the bone marrow

myelomeningocele hernia of the spinal cord and meninges through a defect in the vertebral column. Also known as *meningomyelocele*.

myeloradiculitis inflammation of the spinal cord and nerve roots. **Radicul/o-** means "nerve root."

myeloschisis splitting of the spinal cord

osteomyelitis inflammation of the bone that may extend to the bone marrow

my/o muscle

myalgia muscle pain

myasthenia gravis progressive weakening and fatigue of the skeletal muscles due to abnormalities at the neuromuscular junction. Literally means "a severe muscle weakness."

myocardial infarction (MI) death of a part of the heart muscle due to the lack of oxygen; often the result of an obstruction in the coronary artery preventing the flow of blood to the part. Also known as a *heart attack*.

myocardial ischemia inadequate circulation of blood to the heart muscle (myocardium) due to an obstruction in the coronary artery; may result in an infarction.

myocardiopathy disease of the heart muscle

myocardiorrhaphy to suture the muscle layer of the heart

myocarditis inflammation of the heart muscle

myocardium the thick muscle layer of the heart. Compare with **epicardium**, **endocardium**, and **pericardium**. (See Appendix F, Figure 4.)

myofibril linear, thread-like structure within a muscle cell

myofilament contractile unit of a muscle containing the proteins actin and myosin. Bundles of myofilaments form the myofibril.

myoglobin a pigment in muscle that transports oxygen

myoma benign tumor of muscle tissue

myometrium muscle wall of the uterus

myoneural junction see **neuromuscular junction**

myosarcoma malignant tumor of muscle tissue

myotome instrument used to cut muscle

myotonia see **ton/o**; **myotonia**

myopia
Nearsightedness; an error of refraction in which light rays focus in front of the retina, making vision of near objects clearer than far objects. Compare with **hypermetropia**.

myos/o muscle

myosin a muscle protein responsible for muscle contraction and relaxation. Found in myofilaments.

myositis inflammation of the muscle

myring/o tympanic membrane; eardrum

myringoplasty surgical repair of the eardrum following its rupture, often due to increased pressure from pyogenic material. Also known as *tympanoplasty*.

myringotomy incision of the tympanic membrane for the drainage of pus-filled fluid, which may accumulate in the middle ear during an infection. If not drained, pressure from the fluid may rupture the tympanic membrane.

myx/o mucus

myxedema physical and mental lethargy in adults as a result of decreased metabolic rates due to hyposecretion of thyroxin from the thyroid gland.

Na⁺- K⁺ pump Active transport mechanism that maintains a high sodium ion concentration outside the cell and a high potassium ion concentration inside the cell.

narc/o numbness

*narc*olepsy an uncontrollable desire to sleep during daytime activities

Memory Key: -lepsy means "seizure."

*narc*otic highly addictive drugs used to relieve pain and induce sleep. Examples include: morphine, codeine, opium, heroin, cocaine, and a variety of synthetic drugs.

naris Nostril; plural is *nares.*

nas/o nose

*nas*al pertaining to the nose

*nas*al cavity hollow space of the respiratory system between the nostrils and pharynx; the nasal septum divides the cavity into right and left halves. (See Appendix F, Figure 18.)

*nas*al conchae bony plates on the lateral wall of each nasal cavity; resemble shell-like structures. Also known as *turbinates.*

*nas*al septum wall dividing the nasal cavity in right and left halves; composed of bone and cartilage

*nas*ogastric tube a tube placed into the nose and extending into the stomach for the insertion or withdrawal of substances

*nas*olacrimal duct see **lacrim/o**

*nas*opharynx portion of the pharynx posterior to the nasal cavity

nat/o birth

ante*nat*al before birth referring to the fetus; prenatal

neo*nat*al a newborn infant up to six weeks of age

perinatal the period just before and after birth

postnatal after birth with reference to the newborn. Compare with **postpartum** under **post-**.

prenatal before birth with reference to the fetus; antenatal

natural immunity See **immun/o, immunity**

natural killer cells Leukocytes that attack
cancerous cells and specific body cells that have been infected by viruses.

navicular One of seven bones of the ankle. See **tarsal bones**.

nearsightedness Vision defect resulting in sharp
focus only for objects close to the eye. See **myopia**.

necr/o death

necropsy postmortem examination; autopsy

necrosis death of cells or tissue

necrotic pertaining to tissue or cellular death

negative feedback A mechanism to maintain
homeostasis whereby a stimulus initiates a response that will reverse or reduce the stimulus, thereby stopping the response until the stimulus occurs again. For example, an above-normal blood sugar will result in a release of insulin to decrease the sugar level of the body. Compare with **positive feedback**.

ne/o new

neonatal a newborn up to six weeks of age

neoplasm a new growth; a mass or tumor that can be benign or malignant

nephr/o kidney

hydronephrosis see **hydr/o**

nephroblastoma a malignant neoplasm of the kidney containing embryonic tissue; occurs in children. Also known as *Wilms' tumor*.

nephrolithiasis stones in the kidney

nephrologist specialist in the study of the kidney

nephron structural and functional unit of the kidney that forms urine; consists of the renal corpuscle and renal tubule

nephropathy any disease of the kidney

nephropexy surgical fixation of the kidney to secure a displaced or drooping kidney to its normal position

nephroptosis drooping kidney

nephrosis abnormal condition of the kidney

nephrotomography procedure that utilizes x-rays to produce images of an organ at various depths following injection of a contrast medium. See **tom/o, tomography**.

pyelonephritis inflammation of the kidney and renal pelvis

nerve
A group of neurons that transmits electrical impulses from the central nervous system to other parts of the body.

afferent n.: nerves that carry impulses toward the brain and spinal cord. Also known as *sensory* nerves.

cranial n.: 12 pairs of nerves emerging bilaterally from the brain to stimulate the muscles of the head, neck, and trunk. Included are I Olfactory, II Optic, III Oculomotor, IV Trochlear, V Trigeminal, VI Abducens, VII Facial, VIII Vestibulocochlear, IX Glossopharyngeal, X Vagus, XI Accessory, XII Hypoglossal.

efferent n.: nerves that carry impulses away from the brain and spinal cord. Also known as *motor* nerves.

mixed n.: nerves that have both sensory (afferent) and motor (efferent) fibers.

motor n.: efferent nerves

peripheral n.: nerves located outside the brain and spinal cord.

sensory n.: afferent nerves

spinal n.: 31 pairs of spinal nerves that emerge from the spinal cord. Each pair is named after the portion of the spinal cord from which it extends. The spinal nerves include 8 pairs of cervical nerves (C1 to C8), 12 pairs of thoracic nerves (T1 to T12), 5 pairs of lumbar nerves (T1 to T5), 5 pairs of sacral nerves (S1 to S5), and 1 pair of coccygeal nerves (Co1). Spinal nerves branch into smaller nerves and are generally named after the organs they stimulate.

nerve cells There are two types of nerve cells: neurons, which transmit electrical impulses, and neuroglia, which are supportive and connective in function.

nerve-cell fiber A thin, slender extension of a neuron. Also known as the *axon*. Can be myelinated (wrapped in myelin sheath) or demyelinated (not wrapped in myelin sheath).

nerve impulse The electrical charge in a muscle or nerve when stimulated; an action potential.

nerve tract A group of nerve fibers within the central nervous system that shares a common function; can be sensory (ascending) or motor (descending).

nervous system See **system**.

neurilemma A thin membrane covering the myelin sheath of some axons, especially the peripheral nerves. Also spelled **neurolemma**.

neur/o nerve

neuralgia nerve pain

neuritis inflammation of a nerve

neuroblastoma a malignant tumor arising from neurons

neurogenic shock see **shock**

neuroglia nerve cells that are supportive and connective in function. Neuroglia do not transmit impulses.

neurohormone a hormone secreted by neurons

neurohypophysis posterior pituitary gland. See **-physis**.

neurology the branch of medicine that deals in the study of the nervous system and its disorders

neurolysis destruction of nerve tissue; the freeing of adhesions from around a nerve

neuromuscular junction the point at which a nerve meets a muscle. Also known as the *myoneural junction*.

neurotransmitter a chemical released from nerve endings that acts on a muscle or another nerve causing it to generate its own electrical impulse. There are many neurotransmitters including acetylcholine, norepinephrine, epinephrine, dopamine, seratonin, and GABA (gamma-aminobutyric acid).

neuron A microscopic nerve cell that conducts electrical impulses.

afferent n.: sensory neuron

efferent n.: motor neuron

interneuron: nerve cell that carries impulses between a sensory and motor neuron.

motor (efferent) n: a neuron that transmits impulses away from the brain and spinal cord to muscles and glands, resulting in movement

multipolar n.: see **multi-, multipolar neuron**.

sensory (afferent) n: a neuron that transmits impulses to the brain and spinal cord.

neutr/o neutral

neutrons a particle that has no electrical charge; found in the nucleus of an atom

neutrophil type of white blood cell. See **-phil**.

nevus A skin lesion; plural is nevi. See **mole**, definition (2).

Nissl substance A substance located in the neuron and important in protein synthesis. (See Appendix F, Figure 13.)

nociceptor A sensory receptor that receives pain; located in skin and internal organs.

nocturia Frequent urination at night.

node of Ranvier Constrictions occurring on myelinated nerve fibers. (See Appendix F, Figure 13.)

nodule A solid, elevated skin lesion greater than 1 cm.

nonstriated involuntary muscle A visceral muscle. See **muscle, visceral**.

noradrenaline See **norepinephrine**.

norepinephrine (1) A hormone (noradrenaline) secreted by the adrenal medulla causing vasoconstriction, thereby increasing blood pressure; a catecholamine. (2) A neurotransmitter.

normal flora Bacteria that normally grow in the intestine.

normal sinus rhythm The proper and sequential conduction of electrical impulses through the heart, from the sinoatrial node to the Purkinje fibers.

normochromia Red blood cells of normal color.

nose The anatomical structure located externally on the face and internally as the nasal cavity; functions in smell and respiration.

nucle/o nucleus

nuclease an enzyme that digests nucleic acid

nucleic acid a major substance of chromosomes. There are two types, deoxyribonucleic acids (DNA) and ribonucleic acids (RNA).

nucleolus small circular structure in the cell nucleus that is the site of ribosome creation

nucleoplasm the protoplasm found in the nucleus of the cell. Also known as *karyoplasm*.

nucleus the central portion of the cell important in reproduction, metabolism, and growth

nucleus pulposus the gelatinous central portion of the intervertebral disk surrounded by annulus fibrosus

nulli- none

nulligravida a woman who has never been pregnant

nullipara a woman who has never given birth

nutrient A nourishing substance in food that is used by the body for growth, repair, energy, and metabolism.

nystagmus Oscillatory movement of the eyeball.

ob- facing toward; at the back of; up; completely

obstetrics branch of medicine dealing with the management of women during pregnancy, childbirth and postpartum. **Stetr/o** comes from Latin meaning "midwife."

Memory Key: Literally, **obstetrics** means "a midwife who stands in front of the birthing mother."

occipital lobe back portion of the cerebrum. (See Appendix F, Figure 11.) For a complete listing of lobes see **lob/o, lobes of cerebrum**.

Memory Key: ob- changes to **oc-** before roots starting with **c**.

occlusion closure, as in the closing up of opposing teeth between the upper and lower jaws. See Memory Key under **occipital lobe** above.

occult hidden; occult blood in the stool is completely hidden from view. See Memory Key under **occipital lobe** above.

ocul/o

extraocular pertaining to outside the eye

intraocular pertaining to within the eye

oculomotor nerve sixth cranial nerve responsible for eye movement

oculus dexter (OD) right eye

oculus sinister (OS) left eye

odont/o tooth

endodontist dentist who specializes in the diagnosis and treatment of diseases within the tooth, such as the pulp

odontoid process toothlike projection extending from the second cervical vertebra on which the head rotates. Also known as *dens*.

orthodontist dentist who specializes in the correction of deformed or maloccluded teeth

periodontist specialist in diseases of tissues around the tooth, such as the gums and cementum

olecranon process
A projection extending from the proximal ulna; commonly known as the *elbow*.

olfaction
The sense of smell.

oligo- scanty; few

*oligo*dipsia diminished thirst
*oligo*menorrhea diminished or infrequent menstruation
*oligo*pnea diminished breathing
*oligo*spermia deficient number of spermatozoa
*olig*uria diminished urination

-oma tumor; new growth

Memory Key 1: There are many medical words ending in **-oma** that can be defined easily by analyzing the word and defining the anatomical root to which **-oma** is attached.

Memory Key 2: **-oma** can refer to a benign or malignant growth.

adeno*ma* benign glandular tumor
carcino*ma* malignant tumor of epithelial tissues
chondro*ma* benign tumor of cartilage
hepato*ma* benign or malignant tumor of the liver
osteo*ma* benign tumor of bone
sarco*ma* a broad term used to indicate malignant tumors of connective tissue structures, such as bone (osteosarcoma) and muscle (myosarcoma)

omentum
An extension of the peritoneum from the stomach. Includes the

greater o.: a double fold of peritoneum, extending from the greater curvature of the stomach like an apron, folding upon itself, returning superiorly, and attaching to the transverse colon.

lesser o.: passes from the lesser curvature of the stomach to the liver.

onc/o tumor; swelling; mass

oncogenesis tumor development and formation
oncology the branch of medicine dealing with tumors

onych/o nail

ep**onych**ium structure upon the nail; cuticle

Memory Key: The **i** is dropped from **-epi** as **onych/o** begins with a vowel.

onychomycosis fungal infection of the nail; tinea unguium
par**onych**ia inflammation of tissue around the nail

Memory Key 1: The **a** is dropped from **para-** because **onych/o** starts with a vowel.

Memory Key 2: The suffix **-itis** is not used in this term although the definition is inflammation.

o/o egg

oöcyte egg cell; the developing ovum

Memory Key: The **ö** indicates that each **o** is to be pronounced separately (OH-oh-sight).

oögenesis formation of the ovum. See Memory Key under **oöcyte**.

oöphor/o ovary

oöphororrhagia hemorrhaging from the ovary. See Memory Key under **oöcyte**.
oöphororrhaphy suturing of the ovary. See Memory Key under **oöcyte**.
oöphorosalpingectomy surgical removal of the ovary and fallopian tube. See Memory Key under **oöcyte**.

open fracture A broken bone that pierces the skin; a
compound fracture. (See Appendix F, Figure 20.)

ophthalm/o eye

Memory Key: The root **ophthalm/o** is often spelled incorrectly; remember, there is an **h** on either side of the **t**.

exophthalmos outward protrusion of the eyeball
ophthalmologist specialist in the study of the diagnosis and treatment of medical and surgical eye disorders
ophthalmoscopy process of visually examining the eye; funduscopy

-opia, -opsia visual condition; vision

amblyopia dimmed or reduced vision
diplopia double vision
hemianopsia lack of vision in half the visual field
hypermetropia farsightedness. See **hypermetropia** under **hyper-**.
hyperopia hypermetropia; farsightedness. See **hypermetropia** under **hyper-**.
myopia nearsightedness. See under the term **myopia**.
presbyopia impaired vision due to old age

-opsy process of viewing

autopsy postmortem examination; necropsy. See **auto-, autopsy**.
biopsy microscopic examination of living tissue. See **bi/o, biopsy**.
necropsy autopsy; postmortem examination. See **auto-, autopsy**.

opt/o vision; sight

optic pertaining to vision or sight
optic chiasm the point at which medial fibers of each optic nerve cross in the brain; important for normal vision to occur
optic disc small area of the retina through which the optic nerve passes; it has no rods or cones and thus, does not produce any visual image

optician expert who fills prescriptions for eyeglasses and contact lenses. Opticians are not physicians and do not carry out medical and surgical treatment of eye conditions.

optometrist specialist in the testing of visual function and in the diagnosis and nonsurgical treatment of eye conditions. Optometrists prescribe eyeglasses and contact lenses and are licensed in some areas to prescribe medication. They do not have a degree in medicine.

-or one who; that which

abductor see **abductor** under **ab-**
adductor see **adductor** under **ad-**
donor one who donates
ventilator that which delivers air to the lungs

orbit The bony cavity of the skull that protects and contains the eyeball.

orchid/o, orchi/o testicles; testes

cryptorchidism undescended testicles; see **crypt/o**
orchidectomy surgical excision of the testicle
orchidopexy surgical fixation of the testicle onto the scrotum
orchitis inflammation of the testicle

Memory Key: Orchids, the beautiful flowers, were so named because the double root on these plants resembled little testicles.

organ A collection of tissue types working together to perform a specific function or functions.

organ of Corti Receptors of hearing located in the cochlea of the inner ear.

organelle Microscopic, intracellular structures that have a specific function.

organic compound A compound containing carbon.

organism Any living thing, animal, or plant.

organomegaly
Enlarged internal organs; visceromegaly.

organs of special sense
See **system**.

origin
A term used for muscle attachment to the bone that does not move when the muscle contracts. Compare with **insertion**.

or/o mouth
oral pertaining to the mouth

Memory Key: Do not confuse **oral** with **aural**, meaning "pertaining to the ear," as the pronunciations are similar.

oral cavity body cavity formed by the cheeks, lips, and dental arches. (See Appendix F, Figure 6.)
oropharynx portion of the pharynx behind the mouth

orth/o straight
orthodontics dental specialty dealing with the correction of deformed or maloccluded teeth
orthopedics surgical specialty dealing with the correction and prevention of deformities of the musculoskeletal structures
orthopnea breathing only in the upright position

os bone
os calcis heel bone
os coxa hip bone; plural is os coxae
os pubis pubic bone; one of three bones that fuse together to form the hip bone

os mouth
cervical os the mouthlike opening at the entrance of the cervix uteri

-ose carbohydrate
Memory Key: **-ose** is a suffix indicating the chemical is a carbohydrate.

dextrose monosaccharide known as *glucose*

fructose monosaccharide found in fruit juices and honey; a simple sugar

galactose monosaccharide or simple sugar found in lactose

glucose simple sugar, which is the body's main source of energy; a monosaccharide. Also known as *dextrose*.

lactose disaccharide found in milk

maltose disaccharide found in malt products, used as a sweetener

sucrose disaccharide broken down into glucose and fructose by the action of sucrase

-osis abnormal condition

arthrosis abnormal condition of joints

cyanosis abnormal bluish discoloration of the lips, skin, and mucous membrane due to the lack of oxygen in the blood

hemarthrosis abnormal accumulation of blood in a joint

mycosis any disease caused by a fungus

nephrosis abnormal condition of the kidney

osmosis
The diffusion of water through a semipermeable membrane.

osmotic pressure
Pressure required to terminate the passage of water into a solution through a semipermeable membrane.

osse/o, oss/i bone

osseous pertaining to bone

ossicles tiny bones in the middle ear. Include the malleus, incus, and stapes. Also known as *hammer*, *anvil*, and *stirrup* respectively.

ossification process of bone formation

osteon
The basic unit of structure of compact bone, including the lamellae and Haversian canal.

oste/o bone

endosteum portion of a long bone. See **endo-**.

osteoarthritis see **arthritis**
osteoblast immature bone cell
osteochondritis inflammation of bone and cartilage
osteoclasis surgical fracture or refracture of bone
osteoclast bone cell that breaks down bone
osteocyte mature bone cell
osteogenesis formation of bone
osteogenic sarcoma malignant tumor of bone;
   osteosarcoma
osteomalacia softening of bone
osteomyelitis inflammation of the bone, which may extend
   to the bone marrow
osteopenia decreased bone density
osteoporosis a condition in which bone tissue is lost and not
   replaced, resulting in weakened bones that can fracture more
   easily
osteosarcoma malignant tumor of bone; osteogenic sarcoma
osteotome instrument used to cut bone
osteotomy incision into bone
periosteum portion of a long bone. See **peri-**.

ot/o ear

otalgia earache
otitis media inflammation of the middle ear
otorhinolaryngologist (ENT) specialist dealing with the
   medical and surgical treatment of the ears, nose, and throat

Memory Key: Note that **laryng/o** is the root used in the
medical term, not **pharyng/o**, even though the definition
refers to the ears, nose, and throat.

otorrhea discharge from the ear
otosclerosis middle ear disorder in which the stapes hardens
   against the oval window causing it to become immobile.
   Transmission of sound waves is interrupted resulting in
   deafness.
otoscope instrument used to examine the ear

ovari/o ovary

ovarian cyst see **cyst**

ovariocentesis surgical puncture to remove fluid from the ovary

ovariorrhexis rupture of an ovary

ovary
One of two female gonads (sex glands) that produce hormones and ova. (see Appendix F, Figure 16.)

oviduct
One of two fallopian tubes that conducts an egg from an ovary to the uterus.

ovulation
Rupture of the graafian follicle releasing the ovum into the abdominal cavity. Occurs midway through the menstrual cycle.

ovum
The female egg discharged from the ovary at ovulation. See **gamete**.

oxidation
(1) The process of a substance combining with oxygen. (2) An increase of positive charges in an atom with an accompanying loss of electrons.

ox/o oxygen
anoxia lack or deficiency of oxygen; frequently used inter-changeably with **hypoxia**.

hypoxia oxygen insufficiency. Compare with **anoxia**.

oxi-, oxy- oxygen; sharp; quick
oximeter instrument used to measure the levels of oxygen in the blood

Memory Key: The **-i** spelling is the oldest form—note the use of **-y**

oxygenate to add oxygen to

oxyhemoglobin hemoglobin attached to oxygen

oxytocia quick, rapid labor. Compare with **oxytocin** below.

oxytocin hormone produced by the hypothalamus and stored in the posterior pituitary; stimulates contraction of the uterus during labor, and release of milk by the mammary glands

Memory Key: The suffix **-in** refers to a chemical compound.

pacemaker Specialized tissue in the right atrium that initiates the heart beat. Also known as the *sinoatrial (SA) node*. (See Appendix F, Figure 3.) See **conduction system**.

pachy- thick
pachyderma pathological thickening of the skin
pachymeninges dura mater; see **mening/o**
pachymeningitis inflammation of the pachymeninges

pain receptor See **nociceptor**.

palate Roof the mouth. It separates the oral cavity from the nasal cavity and consists of a bony **hard palate** and a **soft palate** composed of connective tissue

palat/o palate
palatine tonsils see **tonsill/o, tonsils**
palatoplasty surgical reconstruction of the palate to correct a cleft palate
palatorrhaphy suturing of the palate to correct cleft palate. Also known as *staphylorrhaphy*.
palatoschisis congenital cleft or split of the palate due to failure of the palate to fuse during embryonic development. Also known as *cleft palate*.

palpation To feel or to touch lightly with the hands; palpation is one of four techniques used during the physical examination as an aid to diagnosis. The other techniques are inspection (looking), percussion (tapping), and auscultation (listening). Together with palpation, the entire process can be abbreviated IPPA.

palpebr/o eyelid

palpebra eyelid
palpebral pertaining to the eyelid

palpitation
The abnormal, rapid throbbing of the heart of which the patient is consciously aware.

Memory Key: Do not confuse **palpitation** with **palpate**, meaning "to feel."

pan- all

Memory Key: A related English word is *pan*orama, meaning "a view in all directions."

*pan*carditis inflammation of all the structures of the heart
*pan*cytopenia deficiency of all cellular elements of the blood
*pan*hypopituitarism deficiency in all pituitary hormones
*pan*hysterectomy surgical removal of the entire uterus
*pan*sinusitis inflammation of all the paranasal sinuses

pancreas
An organ resembling a fish, lying behind the stomach in the left upper quadrant; has endocrine and exocrine functions. (See Appendix F, Figure 6.)

pancreat/o pancreas

pancreatic **enzymes** substances produced by the exocrine portion of the pancreas. Enzymes include amylase to break down carbohydrates, lipase to break down fats, and a variety of enzymes that break down protein.
pancreatic **juice** exocrine secretions of the pancreas, which include pancreatic enzymes and sodium bicarbonate
pancreatitis inflammation of the pancreas. May be fatal.
pancreatogenic produced by the pancreas

Pap (Papanicolaou) smear
A laboratory test for early detection of cancerous cells, particularly in the cervix uteri.

papill/o nipple

papilla a small, nipple-like elevation, such as the projections on the tongue that contain taste buds

papilledema accumulation of fluid at the optic papilla (disc), caused by increased intracranial pressure

papilloma any benign epithelial tissue; for example warts

papule A lesion characterized by a solid, elevated area of skin; for example, an acne lesion without pus. If the lesion is greater than I cm in diameter, it is called a *nodule*.

para- beside; abnormal; resembling

paracentesis surgical puncture of the peritoneal cavity to remove fluid; abdominocentesis

paralysis loss of sensory or motor function of a part

Memory Key: In the term **paralysis**, **para-** means "abnormal."

parametrium connective tissue extending from the uterus

paranasal sinus see **sinus/o, sinus** definition (1)

paraplegia paralysis of the lower part of the body including both legs

parasympathetic nervous system part of the autonomic nervous system. Consists of nerve fibers that originate in the cranial and sacral areas and end in muscles and glands. Generates nerve impulses that prepare the body for rest and quiet. The parasympathetic system works in conjunction with the sympathetic system.

parathormone parathyroid hormone

parathyroid gland see **gland**

parathyroid hormone (PTH) hormone secreted by the parathyroid gland; regulates blood calcium and phosphate levels. Also known as *parathormone*.

paresthesia abnormal sensation such as burning, itching, or tingling in the absence of external stimulation

Memory Key: The vowel **a** is dropped from **para-** because the root begins with a vowel.

paronychia inflammation of tissue beside the nail. See Memory Key under **onych/o, paronychia**.

parotid gland see **gland**

-para to bear; give birth

multi*para* a woman who has given birth (500 g or 20 weeks gestation) two or more times, whether or not the offspring was alive or dead; written as para II, para III, or PII, PIII, and so on

nulli*para* a woman who has never given birth

primi*para* a woman who has given birth, once only, to an offspring of at least 500 g or 20 weeks gestation, regardless of whether the offspring was alive or dead, or whether it was a single or multiple birth; written para I or PI

secundi*para* a woman who has twice given birth (500 g or 20 weeks gestation), regardless of whether the offspring was alive or dead; written para II or PII

parenchyma The major functional units of an organ. For example, the neurons of the nervous system and the nephrons of the kidney are considered parenchymal tissue.

pariet/o wall

parietal pertaining to the walls of a cavity

parietal bone one of two flat bones that together make up the roof and sides of the skull. (See Appendix F, Figure 19.)

parietal lobe portion of the cerebrum. (See Appendix F, Figure 11.) See **lob/o, lobes of cerebrum**.

parietal membrane serous membrane that lines cavities that do not lead to the exterior, specifically the pericardial, peritoneal, and pleural cavities. Types include:

parietal pericardium: serous membrane that lines the pericardial cavity

parietal peritoneum: serous membrane that lines the peritoneal cavity

parietal pleura: serous membrane that lines the pleural cavity

Parkinson's disease A chronic progressive disorder characterized by bradykinesia, muscular rigidity, slow gait (walk), and resting tremors (twitching while the part is at rest).

paroxysm A sudden attack or recurrence of symptoms of disease.

partial fracture A bone that is incompletely broken; an incomplete fracture.

-partum delivery; birth
ante*partum*; ante *partum* pertaining to the period before birth, referring to the mother
post*partum*; post *partum* pertaining to the period after delivery, referring to the mother

parturition The birth process. See **labor**.

passive acquired immunity See **immunity**.

patch A discolored, unelevated skin lesion of greater than 1 cm.

patell/o patella; kneecap
infra*patellar* pertaining to below the kneecap
patella kneecap. (See Appendix F, Figure 19.)

Memory Key: -a is a noun ending.

patellar reflex. See **reflex**
*patello*pexy surgical fixation of the knee
supra*patellar* pertaining to above the kneecap

patency The state of being wide open.

path/o disease
*path*ogen a substance, such as a microorganism, capable of producing disease
*path*ogenesis development of a disease

pathologist a specialist in the study of disease, its nature, and cause

pathology the branch of medicine dealing with the study of disease, its nature, and cause

pathophysiology the study of diseases as related to body functions

-pathy disease process

Memory Key: -y means "process."

cardiomyopathy any disease process of the heart muscle

encephalomyelopathy any disease process of the brain and spinal cord

lymphadenopathy any disease process of the lymph nodes, particularly enlargement

nephropathy any kidney disease

neuropathy any disease of the nerves

retinopathy any disease of the retina

pector/o chest

angina pectoris chest pain. See **ang-**.

pectoral girdle the bony structure that attaches the upper limbs to the trunk; consists of the clavicle and scapula

ped/o child

pediatrics branch of medicine that deals with the treatment of diseases of children, usually 13 years and under

ped/o foot

pedicle a footlike or stalklike attachment. Also known as a *peduncle*. Literally means "a little foot."

pelv/i pelvis

pelvic cavity space below the abdomen containing the urinary bladder and reproductive organs

pelvic girdle the bony structure that attaches the lower extremities to the trunk; consists of the two hip bones joined anteriorly at the symphysis pubis and posteriorly at the sacrum

pelvic inflammatory disease (PID) bacterial infection extending beyond the cervix uteri

pelvimetry process of measuring pelvic dimensions to determine if the pelvis will allow the passage of the fetus through the birth canal

-penia deficient; decrease

erythrocyto*penia* deficiency in the number of red blood cells; erythropenia

leukocyto*penia* deficiency in the number of white blood cells; leukopenia.

pancyto*penia* deficiency of all cellular elements of the blood

penis The external male sex organ. (See Appendix F, Figure 17.)

pepsin An enzyme secreted by gastric cells that starts the breakdown of protein in the stomach.

pepsinogen The precursor of pepsin; pepsinogen changes into pepsin when it is secreted from gastric cells.

peptic ulcer See **ulcer**.

peptidases Digestive enzymes secreted by the small intestine that convert peptides to amino acids.

peptide bond A chemical bond that links two amino acids in a protein molecule.

per- through

***per*cutaneous** through the skin

percutaneous radiofrequency rhizotomy: a procedure in which percutaneous radio waves are used to alleviate pain in trigeminal neuralgia.

percutaneous transhepatic cholangiography: fluoroscopic examination of the biliary tree following injection of a contrast medium through the skin and liver into the biliary ducts.

percutaneous transluminal angioplasty (PTA): surgical procedure using a balloon-tipped catheter to open a blood vessel blocked by fatty plaques. See *angi/o, angioplasty*.

percutaneous ultrasonic lithotripsy: crushing of kidney stones or gallstones using ultrasound that travels through the skin and onto the stones.

perfusion the passage of fluid through vessels of an organ

percussion Tapping parts of the body to determine the density of underlying structures. Percussion is one of four techniques used during the physical examination as an aid to diagnosis. The other techniques are inspection (looking), palpation (feeling), and auscultation (listening). The entire process can be abbreviated IPPA.

peri- around

perianal pertaining to around the anus

periarthritis inflammation of tissues around a joint

pericardial cavity space between the parietal and visceral pericardium

pericarditis inflammation of the pericardium

pericardium saclike structure surrounding the heart. Compare with **endocardium**, **epicardium**, and **pericardium**. (See Appendix F, Figure 4.) Types include:

parietal p.: serous membrane lining the pericardium.

visceral p.: serous membrane covering the heart. Also known as the *epicardium*.

perichondrium connective tissue that covers all cartilage except the articular cartilage

perilymph fluid around the membranous labyrinth or the inner ear. Compare with **endolymph** under **endo-**.

perimetrium outermost wall of the uterus; one of three walls of the uterus, the others being the myometrium and endometrium

perimysium connective tissue surrounding each fasciculus (muscle bundle) in skeletal muscle. Compare with **endomysium** under **endo** and **epimysium** under **ept**.

perinatal the period just before and after birth with reference to the fetus and newborn respectively

periodontal membrane tissue that anchors a tooth in place

periodontist specialist in diseases of tissues around the tooth, such as the gums and cementum

periosteum structure around the diaphysis of the long bone

peripheral located away from the center or central organ

peripheral nervous system portion of the nervous system outside the brain and spinal cord; includes the nerves and ganglia

perirenal pertaining to around the kidney

peristalsis rhythmic, wavelike muscular contractions that propel the contents through a hollow organ. **-Stalsis** means "contraction."

peritubular capillaries blood capillaries that surround the renal tubule and receive useful materials reabsorbed from the renal filtrate

periungual pertaining to around the nail

perineum
The area between the anus and scrotum in the male and the anus and vulva in the female.

Memory Key: Do not confuse **perineum** with **peritoneum**. The **perineum** is the area around the genital area; the peritoneum is a membrane that lines the abdominal cavity.

peritone/o   peritoneum

peritoneal cavity fluid-filled space between the parietal and visceral peritoneum

peritoneum serous membrane in the abdominal and pelvic cavities. See Memory Key under the term **perineum**. Types include:

parietal p.: lines the abdominal and pelvic cavities.

visceral p.: covers the organs in the abdominal and pelvic cavities.

peritonitis inflammation of the peritoneum. May be fatal.

pernicious anemia See **a(n)-, anemia**.

PET scan The abbreviation for *positron emission tomography*. See **scan**.

petechia Pinpoint hemorrhages in the skin caused by any number of vascular and blood disorders; they are small, flat, and purple.

petit mal seizure See **seizure, absence**

-pexy surgical fixation
blepharopexy surgical fixation of the eyelid
metropexy surgical fixation of the uterus; hysteropexy
nephropexy surgical fixation of the kidney

Peyer's patches Lymphoid tissue on the mucous membrane of the small intestine.

pH A symbol of measure expressing the degree of alkalinity or acidity of a substance. The pH scale extends from 0 to 14 with the value of 7 being neutral. A value lower than 7 is acidic, a value higher than 7 is alkaline (basic).

phac/o, phak/o lens of the eye
aphakia absence of the lens of the eye
phacomalacia softening of the lens of the eye
pseudophakia a condition characterized by the replacement
   of the lens with connective tissue

-phagia eat; swallow
aphagia not eating
dysphagia difficulty swallowing
polyphagia excessive eating

phag/o to eat

phagocyte cells that have the ability to engulf and digest dead and foreign material, such as bacteria

phagocytosis the process in which phagocytes engulf and digest dead and foreign material

phalang/o phalanx

inter*phalang*eal between two phalanges

phalanx

One of the bones of the fingers or toes. Plural is *phalanges*.

Memory Key: So named because each phalanx in a finger or toe is lined up with the others, reminding the Romans of a line of soldiers.

pharyng/o throat; pharynx

***pharyng*eal tonsils** adenoids; see **tonsil**

***pharyng*itis** inflammation of the pharynx

***pharyng*oesophageal sphincter** see **sphincter**

pharynx

The throat; passageway for air and food. (See Appendix F, Figure 18.)

-phasia speech

a*phasia* loss or impairment of speech

dys*phasia* defective speech

phenotype

The appearance of an individual as determined both genetically and environmentally. For example, eye color is determined genetically, but height can be altered environmentally.

phenylalanine hydroxylase

An enzyme necessary to change phenylalanine to tyrosine; lack of this enzyme results in increased phenylalanine in the blood spilling over into the urine. Can also lead to mental retardation. See **phenylketonuria**.

phenylketonuria   The accumulation of phenyl-
ketones in the urine; occurs in infants who are born lacking the
enzyme phenylalanine hydroxylase that is necessary to change
phenylalanine to tyrosine. Lack of this enzyme results in an
increase in blood phenylalanine that eventually spills over into
the urine. **Phenylketonuria** can lead to mental retardation if
not treated with a special diet that excludes phenylalanine.

pheochromocytoma   A tumor of the chromaffin
cells of the adrenal medulla.

-phil love; affinity

baso*phil* type of granular white blood cell that stains readily
   with a basic dye
eosino*phil* type of granular white blood cell that stains readily
   with an acid stain eosin
neutro*phil* type of granular white blood cell that stains readily with a neutral dye. The nucleus is divided into lobes by
   fine threads giving it the appearance of many-shaped nuclei.
   Also known as a *polymorphonuclear leukocyte*.

phimosis   A tightened foreskin that cannot be pulled
back.

phleb/o vein

***phleb*itis** inflammation of a vein
***phleb*ostenosis** narrowing of a vein
***phleb*othrombosis** abnormal condition of clots in a vein
***phleb*otomy** incision into a vein
thrombo*phleb*itis inflammation of a vein with clot formation

phlegm   Thick mucus secreted from the respiratory tract.

-phobia fear

acro*phobia* fear of heights
agora*phobia* fear of crowded places
claustro*phobia* fear of enclosed spaces
photo*phobia* intolerance to light

-phonia

aphonia loss of voice

dysphonia difficulty in speaking

-phoresis transmission; carry

electrophoresis a laboratory test in which substances in a mixture, usually proteins, are separated by an electrical current

phosphodiesterase An enzyme that degrades cyclic adenosine monophosphate (AMP).

phospholipid A lipid that contains phosphoric acid.

phosphorus See **mineral**.

phosphorylation A metabolic process that attaches a phosphate group to an organic molecule or enzyme.

phot/o light

photocoagulation a procedure in which a beam of light from a laser condenses protein material; may be used to repair retinal detachment

photophobia intolerance to light

photoreceptors sensory nerve endings that are stimulated by light; the rods and cones of the retina are photoreceptors

photorefractive keratectomy (PRK) a procedure utilizing an intense beam of light from a laser to remove thin layers of corneal tissue; used to treat farsightedness, nearsighted-ness, and astigmatism

photoretinitis inflammation of the retina due to exposure to intense light

phren/o diaphragm

phrenic nerve peripheral nerves that stimulate the diaphragm

phrenoplegia paralysis of the diaphragm

physi/o nature

physician specialist in the study of medicine who has graduated from a recognized medical school and is licensed to practice by the appropriate authority

physiology the branch of science dealing with the function of cells, tissues, and organs

physiotherapy treatment by physical means such as exercise and massage

-physis to grow

adenohypophysis another name for the anterior pituitary. So called because the anterior pituitary is composed of glandular epithelial cells that produce and secrete hormones.

diaphysis the shaft of the long bone

epiphysis bulbous portion at the proximal and distal ends of the long bone

hypophysis pituitary gland. (See Appendix F, Figure 7.)

neurohypophysis another name for the posterior pituitary. So called because the posterior pituitary is composed of nerve cell fibers that store and secrete hormones produced in the hypothalamus.

pia mater The innermost membrane covering the brain and spinal cord. See **mening/o**; **meninges**. (See Appendix F, Figure 12.)

pil/o hair

pilonidal cyst an enclosed sac in the sacral region, usually containing a cluster of hairs. **Nid/o** means "nest."

pineal gland See **gland**.

pink eye See **conjunctivitis**.

pinna The flap of the ear; auricle. (See Appendix F, Figure 14.)

pinocytosis The process by which small quantities of fluid are taken into the cell.

pisiform One of eight carpal bones. See **carpal bones** under **carp/o**.

pituitary gland See **gland**.

placenta The organ formed in the uterus during pregnancy; site of exchange of substances between fetal and maternal blood.

plane An imaginary line that cuts the body or body parts in specific ways. Examples include:

coronal p.: frontal plane.

frontal p.: cuts the body into front and back. Also known as *coronal plane*.

horizontal p.: transverse plane

midsagittal p.: cuts the body into right and left equal portions.

sagittal p.: cuts the body into right and left unequal portions. See Memory Key under **suture, sagittal**.

transverse p.: cuts the body into inferior and superior portions, which may be unequal. Also known as *horizontal plane*.

plantar The sole of the foot; for example, plantar warts are benign skin growths appearing on the sole of the foot.

plantar flexion The bending of the foot at the ankle joint toward the sole

plantar reflex See **reflex**.

-plasm plasma

cyto*plasm* protoplasm of the cell located between the cell membrane and nucleus

neo*plasm* new and abnormal growth or mass of tissue

plasma The fluid portion of the blood in which blood cells float.

plasma cell A cell derived from B lymphocytes that produce antibodies.

plasma membrane See **cell membrane**.

plasma proteins Proteins that circulate in the liquid portion of blood. Includes clotting factors, albumin, and globulin.

-plasty surgical repair; surgical reconstruction

arthro*plasty* surgical reconstruction of a joint. See **arthr/o, arthroplasty**.
cheilo*plasty* surgical reconstruction of a lip
orchido*plasty* surgical reconstruction of a testicle
rhino*plasty* surgical reconstruction of the nose; "nose job"

platelet A blood cell responsible for clotting. Also known *thrombocyte*. **Platelet** literally means "little plate."

-plegia paralysis

di*plegia* paralysis affecting similar parts on both sides of the body
hemi*plegia* paralysis of either the right or left half of the body
mono*plegia* paralysis of one limb
para*plegia* paralysis of the lower part of the body including both legs. **Para-** means "abnormal."
quadri*plegia* paralysis of all four limbs

pleurisy Inflammation of the pleura.

pleur/o pleura

pleura serous membrane in the thoracic cavity. Includes:
  parietal p.: serous membrane lining the thoracic cavity
  visceral p.: serous membrane covering the lungs
*pleuro*centesis surgical puncture of the pleural cavity to remove fluid. Also known as *thoracocentesis* or *pleuracentesis*.
pleural cavity fluid-filled space between the parietal and visceral pleura

*pleur*al **effusion** escape of fluid into the pleural cavity

*pleur*algia pain in the pleura

plexus network A network of nerves or capillaries.
Examples include:

brachial p.: a network of nerves located in the neck and upper arm from which spinal nerves emerge to stimulate the skin and muscles of the arm and hand.

cervical p.: a network of nerves located in the neck region from which the spinal and phrenic nerves emerge.

choroid p.: a network of capillaries in the ventricles of the brain that filter blood, producing cerebrospinal fluid as the filtrate.

lumbar p.: a network of nerves located in the lower back from which nerves emerge to stimulate the lower abdomen, hip, and leg region.

sacral p.: a network of nerves that emerge from the sacral area to stimulate the leg.

Meissner's p.: a network of nerves situated in the submucosa of the small intestine.

plica circulares Circular folds in the small intestine
that increase the surface area for absorption. **Plica** means "fold."

-pnea breathing

a*pnea* no breathing

brady*pnea* slow breathing

dys*pnea* painful breathing

eu*pnea* normal breathing

hyper*pnea* abnormal increase in the depth and rate of breathing

oligo*pnea* infrequent breathing resulting in a reduction of air entering the lungs

ortho*pnea* breathing only in the upright position

tachy*pnea* fast breathing

pneum/o lung; air

pneumoconiosis any number of abnormal conditions characterized by the accumulation of dust particles in the lung.
Coni/o means "dust." Pneumoconioses are named after the
type of dust that is inhaled. Foe example:

anthracosis: the result of inhalation of coal dust in coal
mining (black lung disease) For example:

asbestosis: the result of inhalation of asbestos dust particles in construction and shipbuilding

silicosis: the result of inhalation of silica dust in rock or
glass grinding

pneumonectomy partial or total removal of the lung

pneumonia inflammation of the lung. Also known as *pneu-
monitis.*

Memory Key: Although the suffix **-itis** is not used, **pneumonia** means "inflammation of the lung."

pneumopleuritis inflammation of the lung and pleura

pneumorrhagia pulmonary hemorrhage

pneumothorax air in the pleural cavity

-poiesis, -poietin formation

erythro*poiesis* formation of red blood cells

erythro*poietin* a hormone in the kidney that stimulates the
production of red blood cells

Memory Key: The suffix **-in** means "a chemical compound."

hemato*poiesis* formation of blood cells

poikilocytosis Variation in shape of red blood cells in
the blood. **Poikil/o** means "variation" or "irregular."

polarization Distribution of ions of opposite charge
on either side of a cell membrane. In a resting muscle cell or
neuron, potassium ions are more abundant inside the cell, are
more abundant outside the cell, giving the membrane a
negative charge inside and a positive charge outside.

poliomyelitis Viral inflammation of the gray matter of the spinal cord affecting motor function, often resulting in disabling paralysis. Commonly known as *polio*.

poly- many

*poly*adenoma tumor of many glands

*poly*cystic ovary ovary infiltrated by many cysts. See **cyst**.

*poly*cythemia increase in the total red cell mass in the blood

*poly*dactylism a congenital defect characterized by having more than the normal number of fingers or toes

*poly*dipsia excessive thirst

*poly*morphonuclear leukocytes granular leukocytes that have a nucleus divided into lobes by fine threads making it look as if there are many shaped nuclei. Also known as a *neutrophil*.

*poly*neuritis inflammation of many nerves

*poly*phagia excessive eating

*poly*peptide a chain of two or more amino acids, not yet a specific protein

*poly*saccharide a large carbohydrate that consists of many monosaccharides bonded into a long chain. Examples include glycogen and starch.

*poly*thelia the occurrence of more than one nipple on a breast

*poly*uria frequent urination

polyp A papilloma; a benign tumor (which may be precancerous) of epithelial tissue arising from the mucous membrane and extending into the body cavity; common in the nose and rectum. Polyps can be described as:

pedunculated p.: attached to the mucous membrane by a little foot.

sessile p.: has a broad base attachment.

pons One of three structures making up the brain stem. (See Appendix F, Figure 11.) The word **pons** means "bridge." The pons bridges the midbrain and medulla oblongata.

popliteal Pertaining to the back of the knee.

pores Minute openings.

portal circulation A process in which the blood circulates through two capillary beds instead of one before returning through veins back to the heart. In hepatic portal circulation, blood passes through the capillaries of a digestive organ and the liver before returning to the heart.

positive feedback A process in which a stimulus initiates a response that increases the output of that stimulus. For example, uterine contractions during childbirth stimulate increasingly strong contractions. Compare with **negative feedback**.

positron emission tomography (PET scan) A diagnostic procedure utilizing a radioactive substance and a gamma camera. See **scan**.

post- after

*post*ganglionic nerve fiber the axon of the sympathetic and parasympathetic neuron that is situated after the ganglion and extends to a muscle or gland. Compare with **preganglionic nerve fiber**.

*post*mortem examination inspection of the body after death. See **auto-, autopsy**.

*post*natal pertaining to the period after birth with reference to the newborn

*post*partum pertaining to the period after delivery with reference to the mother

*post*prandial after meals

*post*synaptic cell a cell situated after the synapse, thereby receiving information after the synapse has been crossed

*post*synaptic potential a process in which membrane polarization is either increased or decreased in a postsynaptic cell, caused by the release of neurotransmitters from a presynaptic cell

poster/o situated behind

posterior toward the back of the body or behind an organ; opposite of **anterior**.

posterior **cavity** space located behind the lens of the eye filled with vitreous humor

posterior **chamber** portion of the anterior cavity of the eye between the iris and lens filled with aqueous humor

posterior **column** posterior portion of white matter on either side of the spinal cord. Also known as the *dorsal column*.

posterior **horn** posterior projection of gray matter of the spinal cord. Also known as the *dorsal horn*.

posterior **pituitary gland** see **gland**

posterior **root** one of two roots by which a spinal nerve is attached to the spinal cord. Emerging from the union between the anterior and posterior root is the spinal nerve. Also known as the *dorsal root*.

posteroanterior from the back to the front. In radiology, the posteroanterior (PA) position refers to x-rays that are projected through the body structure from the back to the front.

potassium See **mineral**.

Pott's fracture A fracture involving the distal fibula and medial malleolus. (See Appendix F, Figure 20.)

pouch of Douglas See **cul-de-sac of Douglas**.

pre- before

precancerous a mass of tissue that is not, but may become, malignant

precursor a chemical substance from which another substance is formed

preganglionic nerve fiber the axon of the sympathetic and parasympathetic neuron that is situated before the ganglion; it extends from the central nervous system to the autonomic ganglion where it synapses with a postganglionic neuron. Compare with **postganglionic nerve fiber**.

premenstrual syndrome (PMS) physical and emotional distress occurring in a cyclical pattern related to the menstrual cycle; may include symptoms such as irritability, depression, edema, and fatigue

prenatal pertaining to before birth with reference to the newborn

presynaptic cell a cell carrying electrical impulses toward the synapse; a nerve cell occurring before the synapse

prepuce
The foreskin; usually refers to the excess skin around the penis, although there is a female prepuce covering the clitoris.

presby- old

presbycusis diminished hearing due to old age

presbyopia impaired vision due to old age

prime mover
The muscle that is the most important in producing a specific movement.

primi- first

primigravida a woman pregnant for the first time

primipara a woman who has given birth, once only, to an offspring of at least 500 g or 20 weeks gestation, regardless of whether it is alive or dead, or whether it was a single or multiple birth; written para I or PI

P-R interval
The measurement of the period of time that impulses take to reach the ventricles from the atria.

pro- before; in front of

process a projection from a structure. For example:
   bony p.: part of a bone rising above the level of its surroundings; an outgrowth of bone –
   ciliary p.: hairlike structures extending from the ciliary body

procidentia uteri see **prolapse, third-degree**. **Cidentia** means "to fall."

prodrome symptom or symptoms occurring before the onset of disease. For example, chest pain, tiredness, and shortness of breath are prodromal symptoms of a heart attack.

prognathism abnormal protrusion of the lower jaw. The root *gnath/o* means "jaw."

prognosis prediction of the outcome of the disease

prolapsed uterus a uterus that has slipped downward through the vaginal canal, out of its normal position; displaced uterus. Types include:

first-degree p.: uterus and cervix project through the vaginal canal but not through the introitus.

second-degree p.: uterus is displaced into the vaginal canal with the cervix protruding through the introitus.

third-degree p.: uterus and cervix project through the introitus. Also known as *procidentia uteri*.

prophase first stage of mitosis in which the chromosomes become apparent, the nuclear membrane disappears, and the centrioles begin to migrate

prophylaxis prevention of disease; care given to guard against disease. For example, cleaning and flossing the teeth guards against tooth decay.

protraction to draw out; extension or protrusion

progesterone
A female steroid hormone from the ovaries, adrenal cortex, and placenta; prepares the endometrium for the fertilized egg.

progestin
The name given to progesterone occurring both naturally and synthetically.

prolactin
A hormone produced by the anterior pituitary to stimulate breast development and the formation of milk during pregnancy.

pronation
(1) The act of turning the palms backward or downward. (2) The act of lying face down on the abdomen. Compare with **supination**.

prone (1) Lying on the abdomen, face down. A common phrase on an operative report is, "with the patient in the prone position." (2) Palms are turned downward or backward.

proprioception Position sense; body awareness.

proprioceptor Sensory receptors responding to the movement and position of body parts. Proprioceptors are found in muscles, tendons, joints, and the inner ear.

prostaglandins Hormone-like substances secreted by most cells with a wide variety of functions.

Memory Key: Prostaglandins are so named because they were originally and incorrectly thought to be exclusively produced by the *prostate* gland.

prostate gland See **gland**.

prostat/o prostate gland

prostatectomy surgical removal of the prostate. Types include:

  perineal p.: removal of the prostate through an incision in the perineum

  suprapubic p.: removal of the prostate through an abdominal incision above the pubis

  transurethral resection of the prostate (TURP): partial removal of the prostate by passing the cutting instrument through the urethra. No incision is made into the abdominal cavity.

prostatic **hypertrophy, benign (BPH)** benign enlargement of the prostate gland, usually occurring in men over 50 years of age

prosthesis An artificial body part that replaces a missing or worn-out structure, such as an artificial limb.

prote/o protein

protease an enzyme that aids in the breakdown of protein

Memory Key: The suffix **-ase** is a noun suffix referring to enzyme.

protein an organic compound made up of amino acids

Memory Key: The suffix **-in** is a noun suffix referring to a chemical substance.

proteinuria protein in the urine; albuminuria

prothrombin
A clotting factor converted to thrombin in the chemical clotting process; a substance necessary for blood clotting to occur.

proton
A subatomic particle found in the nucleus of an atom that has a positive electrical charge.

protoplasm
A thick, transparent glue-like substance that makes up the necessary material of all animal and plant cells.

proximal
Toward or nearest the point of origin of a structure, or nearest the point of attachment to the trunk. Opposite of **distal**. For example, the stomach is proximal to the intestines, as the mouth is the point of origin. The elbow is proximal to the wrist, as the elbow is closest to the point of attachment to the trunk.

pruritus
Itching.

pseud/o false; something similar but not quite; not of the true type

pseudocyesis a psychiatric disorder in which the patient has all the signs of pregnancy, such as weight gain, stoppage of menses, and morning sickness, but is not pregnant

pseudocyst a dilatation that looks like a cyst but does not contain the material to properly classify it as a cyst

pseudomembrane a layer that looks like membrane but is not; may form in some types of respiratory conditions making breathing difficult

pseudophakia replacement of the lens with connective tissue

psoriasis One of the most common skin conditions, characterized by silvery scales, papules, and plaques. Cause is unknown.

psych/o mind

psychiatry branch of medicine dealing with the diagnosis, treatment, and prevention of mental illness

psychiatrist specialist in the study of psychiatry

psychology the science that deals with normal and abnormal mental processes that have an effect on behavior

psychologist specialist in the study of psychology

psychosis a major psychiatric disorder in which the patient has lost touch with reality

psychosomatic pertaining to a mind-body relationship; physical conditions of mental or emotional origin

ptosis Downward displacement of a body part from its normal position.

-ptosis drooping; sagging; downward displacement

blepharoptosis drooping of the eyelid due to weakness of the eyelid muscles

nephroptosis drooping of the kidney

Memory Key: **Ptosis** can stand by itself as a noun or it can be used as a suffix attached to a root word.

ptyal/o starch

ptyalin an enzyme found in the saliva that breaks down starch

ptyalism excessive secretion of saliva

-ptysis spitting

hemoptysis spitting up or coughing up of blood from the respiratory tract

pub/o pubis; pubic bone

pubic bone one of three bones making up the os coxa, the other two bones being the ilium and ischium. Also known as *os pubis*.

pudendum External genitalia especially of the female; includes the labia majora, labia minora, mons pubis, clitoris, and Bartholin's glands. Also known as the *vulva*.

pulmon/o lung

*pulmon*ary **artery** artery carrying deoxygenated blood from the right ventricle of the heart to the lungs

*pulmon*ary **circulation** the movement of blood from the heart through the lungs to become oxygenated

*pulmon*ary **edema** accumulation of fluid in the interstitial spaces of the lung

*pulmon*ary **embolism** a clot having wandered into the pulmonary artery, thereby obstructing circulation. See **embolus** under **bol/o**.

*pulmon*ary **function test (PFT)** various tests of lung performance. Include:

expiratory reserve volume (ERV): the volume of air that can be forced from the lungs above normal expiration.

inspiratory reserve volume (IRV): the volume of air that can be forced into the lungs above normal inspiration.

residual volume (RV): the volume of air remaining in the lung following maximal exhalation.

tidal volume (TV): the volume of air taken into the lungs on normal inspiration and expiration.

total lung capacity (TLC): the total volume of air the lungs can hold.

*pulmon*ary **perfusion scan** diagnostic procedure utilizing a radioactive substance and gamma camera. See **scan**.

*pulmon*ary **semilunar valve** see **valve**

*pulmon*ary **ventilation scan** diagnostic procedure utilizing a radioactive substance and gamma camera. See **scan**.

*pulmon*ary **vein** veins carrying oxygenated blood from the lungs to the heart

pulp cavity The hollow structure inside the tooth containing blood vessels and nerves.

pulse The alternating, rhythmical contraction and expansion of the arterial wall in time to the heartbeat. (See

Appendix F, Figure 5.) Pulses can be felt at the following points throughout the body:

brachial p.: arm at the depression anterior to the elbow
carotid p.: neck
dorsalis pedis p.: dorsum of the foot
femoral p.: top of thigh at the groin
popliteal p.: at the knee
radial p.: wrist
temporal p.: temples

punct/o point

punctum the most common punctum is the tiny point in the medial corner of each eye through which tears flow to the lacrimal sac. Plural is *puncta*.

pupil The dark opening of the eye surrounded by the iris through which light rays pass. (See Appendix F, Figure 15.)

pupillary reflex See **reflex**.

Purkinje fibers Part of the independent electrical system of the heart. See **conduction system**. (See Appendix F, Figure 3.)

purpura Small hemorrhages of up to 1 cm in diameter into tissue and mucous membranes. Types include petechiae and ecchymoses.

pus Yellowish-white matter produced by pyogenic bacteria such as staphylococci, streptococci, gonococci, or pneumococci.

pustule A small, elevated skin lesion containing pus.

P waves See **waves**.

pyel/o renal pelvis; dilated upper segment of the ureter

pyelocaliectasis dilatation of the renal pelvis and calices
pyelogram x-ray of the urinary tract. See **ur/o: excretory urogram**; and **retrograde urogram**.

pyelonephritis inflammation of the renal pelvis and kidney

pylor/o pylorus

pyloric sphincter circular muscle in the distal stomach. See
sphincter.

pyloric stenosis narrowing of the pyloric sphincter

pyloromyotomy incision into the pyloric sphincter

pylorospasm sudden, violent, contraction of the pyloric
sphincter. Pyloromyotomy may be performed to relieve the
spasm.

pylorus The narrow opening in the distal stomach leading to
the duodenum. (See Appendix F, Figure 6.)

Memory Key: The suffix **-us** is a noun ending.

py/o pus

empyema accumulation of pus in a body cavity, usually the
thoracic cavity

pyoderma any pus-producing disease of the skin

pyogenic bacteria that produces pus, such as staphylococci,
streptococci, gonococci, or pneumococci

pyosalpinx pus in the fallopian tube

pyothorax pus in the pleural cavity

pyuria pus in the urine

pyrexia High body temperature; fever.

Q

quadri- four Quadreceps have four heads or divisions.

quadriceps femoris anterior muscles of the upper leg composed of four smaller muscles (rectus femoris, vastus lateralis,

vastus medialis and vastus intermedius) that work together to extend the leg. Often referred to as *quadriceps*.

***quadri*plegia** paralysis of all four limbs

QRS waves See **wave**.

rachi/o spine; vertebral column

***rachi*odynia** pain in the vertebral column

***rachi*schisis** congenital splitting of the vertebral column. See **spina bifida**.

***rachi*tis** inflammation of the spine

radiation Emission of certain radioactive elements.

radiation therapy The use of ionizing radiation for diagnostic and therapeutic purposes.

radicul/o nerve root

***radicul*itis** inflammation of the nerve root

radi/o radius

***radi*al artery** blood vessel that provides the radius with oxygenated blood

***radi*al nerve** part of the brachial plexus that stimulates the wrist and hand

***radi*ocarpal joint** union between the radius and the bones of the wrist

radi/o x-rays

radioactive substance capable of emitting radiant energy

radioimmunoassay (RIA) a laboratory test that combines the use of radioactive chemicals and antibodies to detect minute quantities of substance in a patient's blood

radioisotope radioactive forms of elements, such as technetium, technetium-99m, gallium-67, carbon-13, xenon-133, and iodine-131. Radioisotopes are used in nuclear medicine. They are injected, swallowed, or inhaled. A specialized camera, called a gamma camera, detects the radioisotope as it accumulates in the body area being studied. An image of the area is then produced and recorded. Also known as *radionuclide*.

radiolucent structures that permit the passage of x-rays; they appear black on an x-ray film. For example, air in the lungs.

radionuclide see **radioisotope**

radiopaque structures that obstruct the passage of x-rays; they appear white on an x-ray film. For example, bony structures.

radiopharmaceutical combination of a drug or chemical with a radioisotope. Each radiopharmaceutical is intended to concentrate in a specific body organ. With the radioisotope giving off radiation, the organ can be imaged with a gamma camera. For example: technetium-99m pertechnetate.

radius The lateral bone of the lower arm; one of two bones of the lower arm, the other being the ulna. (See Appendix F, Figure 19.)

Memory Key: The radius was so named because the Romans felt the bone resembled the spoke of a wheel.

rales Abnormal crackling sounds made by air passing through bronchi congested with thick mucous secretions.

ramus A branch from a larger structure such as a nerve, bone, or vessel.

Raynaud's syndrome A disease of the peripheral vascular system characterized by spasmodic contraction of the arterioles of the fingers and toes, cutting off circulation to these areas.

re- back

reflux a backward flow; regurgitation

repolarization the restoration of electrical charges on either side of the membrane to its resting state following depolarization. Compare with **depolarization** under **de-**.

resection the removal of an organ or structure either partially or completely

retraction the act of drawing back, such as the retraction of tissue from the operative site to provide a clear surgical field

retractor instrument used to hold back structures that would obscure an operative field

receptor A sensory nerve ending that receives a nervous stimulus.

recessive gene A gene that is responsible for a characteristic that is expressed only if two genes for it are present.

recombinant DNA Artificially constructed DNA made by inserting lengths of DNA from different sources.

rect/o rectum

rectocele hernia or displacement of the rectum onto the vaginal wall

rectouterine pertaining to the rectum and uterus

rectouterine pouch see **cul-de-sac of Douglas**

rectum lower portion of the large intestine

red blood cell (RBC) An erythrocyte; a mature blood cell containing hemoglobin to transport oxygen.

red bone marrow Tissue found in developing long bones of children; in the adult, red bone marrow is found in ribs, vertebrae, pelvic bone, and sternum.

red muscles Darker-colored muscle tissue composed mainly of muscle fibers that contract slowly (slow-twitch muscle fibers); these muscle fibers are red because they contain large amounts of iron-containing substances giving the muscle a reddish appearance.

reduction (1) The repair of a fracture, hernia, or dislocation. (2) Gain of electrons by an atom or molecule.

referred pain Pain felt in parts other than the place of origin.

reflex An involuntary response to a stimulus. Types of reflexes include:

abdominal r.: light scratching or itching of abdominal skin causes contraction of abdominal muscles.

Achilles r.: tapping of the Achilles tendon causes plantar flexion of the foot. Also known as *ankle jerk*.

ankle jerk: see Achilles reflex.

Babinski's r.: an abnormal response to the plantar reflex. See **plantar reflex** below.

corneal r.: stimulation of the cornea results in closing of the eyelids.

deep tendon r.: tapping of the tendon results in the involuntary contraction of its muscle. Examples includes the Achilles and patellar reflexes. Abbreviated DTR.

gag r.: touching the back of the pharynx results in retching (trying to vomit).

gastroesophageal r.: backward flow of gastric contents into the esophagus. Also known as *heartburn*.

knee jerk: see **patellar reflex**.

patellar r.: tapping the patellar ligament results in the lower leg extending. Also known as *knee jerk*.

plantar r.: stroking the sole of the foot results in flexion of the toes. The abnormal response to the plantar reflex is Babinski's reflex, which is dorsiflexion of the great toe when the sole of the foot is stimulated. This reflex is normal in newborns and children up to two years of age, but in others it is a sign of central nervous system disorder.

pupillary r.: exposure of the retina to bright light results in constriction of the pupil of the eye.

superficial r.: touching or irritation of the skin results in a withdrawal reflex.

reflex arc
The pathway traveled by a nerve impulse to produce a reflex action. Includes a sensory receptor, sensory neuron, integration centers in the brain and spinal cord, motor neuron, and effector organ, such as a muscle or gland.

refraction
The bending of light rays. Light rays are refracted through eye structures to focus simultaneously, and at the same point, on the retina.

remission
Lessening of the severity of symptoms. Opposite is *exacerbation*.

renin
An enzyme that catalyzes the formation of angiotensin I from plasma protein.

renin-angiotensin mechanism
A series of chemical reactions initiated by a decrease in blood pressure that stimulates the kidneys to secrete the enzyme renin.

ren/o kidney

Memory Key: The root **ren/o** is usually used in terms dealing with structure.

perirenal fat fat surrounding the outside of the kidney; functions to support the kidney

renal calculi kidney stones

renal capsule one of three covers surrounding the outside of the kidney. The other coverings include perirenal fat and renal fascia.

renal columns tissue of the renal cortex extending between the renal pyramids

renal cortex the outermost area of the internal kidney

renal erythropoietic factor an enzyme found in the kidney that catalyzes the formation of the hormone erythropoietin from plasma protein

renal fascia thin layer of tissue surrounding the kidney serving to support the kidney. Also known as *Gerota's fascia*.

renal medulla the innermost area of the internal kidney made up of the renal pyramids

renal pelvis upper dilated portion of the ureter

renal pyramids triangular tissue of the renal medulla that are separated by renal columns

renal tubule nonvascular part of the nephron consisting of a proximal convoluted tubule, loop of Henle, distal convoluted tubule, and collecting duct; site of tubular reabsorption and tubular secretion

replication The making of an exact copy of DNA during the early stages of mitosis.

reproductive system See **system**.

residual volume (RV) See **pulmonary function test**.

respiration The exchange of oxygen (O_2) and carbon dioxide (CO_2) in the body.

    external r.: involves breathing and the exchange of gases between the air in the lungs and the blood in the pulmonary capillaries.

    internal r.: the exchange of oxygen and carbon dioxide between blood capillaries and tissue cells; oxygen is passed from the blood into the cells and carbon dioxide passes from the cells into the blood.

respiratory distress syndrome (RDS)
A respiratory problem of premature newborns. See **hyaline membrane disease**.

respiratory system   See **system**.

resting membrane potential   The difference in electrical charges on either side of a cell's membrane when the cell is not stimulated; a negative charge inside the cell and a positive charge outside the cell.

reticul/o network

reticular **fiber** immature connective tissue fibers found in such organs as glands, lymph nodes, and skin

reticular **formation** network of cells and fibers in the brain stem playing an important function in the sleep-wake cycle

reticulocyte an immature stage in red blood cell formation

Memory Key: The reticulocyte is so named because its cytoplasm contains a network of fine threadlike material.

*reticulo***endothelial system** see **system**

retinaculum   A wide membranous structure that holds an organ or structure in place, such as the retinaculum at the distal ends of each limb that holds tendons in place when muscles contract.

retin/o retina

retina the inner layer of the eye containing the rods and cones

retinopathy any disease of the retina

retinoschisis splitting of the retina

retinal detachment separating of the retina from the underlying tissue; retinal detachment is more severe than retinoschisis

retr/o back

retroflexion bending back of an organ or part; a retroflexed uterus describes the body of the uterus bending backward toward the rectum

retrograde to flow back

> **retrograde pyelogram:** x-ray of the urinary system. See **ur/o, retrograde urogram**.
>
> **retrograde urogram:** x-ray of the urinary system. See **ur/o, retrograde urogram**.

retroperitoneal situated behind the peritoneum

retroversion the tilting backward of an organ; a retroverted uterus describes the uterus tilting backward toward the rectum

rhabd/o striated; striped

rhabdomyoma benign tumor of striated muscle, such as cardiac and skeletal muscles

rhabdomyosarcoma malignant tumor of striated muscle, such as cardiac and skeletal muscles

rheumatic heart disease A streptococcal infection causing carditis or pancarditis; may lead to valvular insufficiency.

rheumatoid arthritis See **arthritis**.

rheumatologist A specialist in the study and treatment of connective tissue structures, such as joints, muscles, tendons, and fibrous tissue.

Rh factor An antigen normally found on red blood cells of certain individuals said to be Rh positive. *Rh negative* means the individual does not have the Rh antigen.

rhin/o nose

rhinencephalon portion of the cerebral cortex associated with smell

rhinitis inflammation of the mucous membrane of the nose

rhinoplasty surgical reconstruction of the nose; "nose job"

rhinorrhea discharge from the nose

rhinorrhagia nose bleed; epistaxis

rhinotomy incision into the nose

rhiz/o root

rhizolysis a procedure in which percutaneous radio waves are used to break down part of the trigeminal nerve in an attempt to alleviate the intense pain caused by trigeminal neuralgia. Also known as *percutaneous radiofrequency rhizotomy*.

rhizotomy incision into a spinal root to interrupt sensory nerve impulses; performed to relieve intractable pain

rhodopsin
The chemical essential for vision in dim light; chemical in the rods of the retina that break down in light, producing stimulation of the sensory nerve.

RhoGam
The trade name for the Rh(D) antibody administered to an Rh-negative mother after delivery of an Rh-positive baby to prevent hemolytic disease of the newborn in future pregnancies; it will destroy any Rh-positive red blood cells that have entered the mother's body. The dose must be repeated after each delivery.

rhonchus
A rale characterized by snoring-like sounds made by air passing through bronchi congested with thick mucous secretions. Plural is *rhonchi*.

rib
One of 24 curved bones forming part of the thoracic cage. There are 12 pairs of ribs classified into the following categories:

true r.: the first seven pairs of ribs that join the sternum anteriorly through direct attachment via costal cartilage, that is, one costal cartilage attaches one rib to the sternum.

false r.: rib pairs eight to twelve; the cartilage of pairs eight to ten join the costal cartilage of the seventh rib anteriorly instead of each attaching directly to the sternum. Rib pairs eleven and twelve do not attach to the sternum at all and are called floating ribs.

floating r.: rib pairs (eleven and twelve) that do not attach to the sternum.

ribonucleic acid (RNA) A nucleic acid important in intracellular protein synthesis.

rod A photoreceptor in the retina of the eye sensitive to dim light; contains rhodopsin.

rotation The circular movement around an axis.

-rrhage, -rrhagia abnormal or excessive flow; bursting forth

gastrorrhagia bleeding from the stomach
hemorrhage bleeding; abnormal flow of blood
pneumorrhagia bleeding from the lung
splenorrhagia bleeding from the spleen
urethrorrhagia bleeding from the urethra

-rrhaphy suture; to sew

cheilorrhaphy to suture the lip
colporrhaphy to suture the vagina
episiorrhaphy to suture the vulva and perineum. See **episi/o**.
fasciorrhaphy suturing of the fascia
gastrorrhaphy to suture a stomach wound
herniorrhaphy surgical repair of a hernia
hysterorrhaphy to suture the uterus
myocardiorrhaphy to suture the muscular layer of the heart
splenorrhaphy to suture a wound of the spleen

-rrhea flow; discharge

dacryorrhea excessive flow of tears

diarrhea bowel movements that are too frequent and loose
galactorrhea see **galact/o**
rhinorrhea discharge from the nose
otorrhea discharge from the ear
seborrhea increased discharge of sebum from the sebaceous
  gland

-rrhexis rupture

amniorrhexis ruptured amnion
arteriorrhexis ruptured artery
cardiorrhexis ruptured heart
ovariorrhexis ruptured ovary
splenorrhexis ruptured spleen

rugae Folds of mucous membrane on the walls of the
stomach, urinary bladder, and vagina that increase the surface
area of that organ.

saccule Membranous sac of the inner ear responsible for
balance.

sacr/o sacrum

sacrococcygeal pertaining the sacrum and coccyx (tailbone)
sacroiliac joint union between the sacrum and the ilium (hip
  bone); iliosacral joint
sacrum bone of lower back. See **vertebra**.

sagittal plane See **plane**.

sagittal suture The immovable joint in the skull. See
suture.

saline solution A solution of salt and distilled water that has many uses, including hydration following the loss of body fluid.

salivary gland See **gland**.

salping/o fallopian tube; eustachian tube

*salping*itis inflammation of the fallopian tube

*salping*ogram X-ray record of the fallopian tubes following injection of a contrast medium

*salping*ography process of recording the fallopian tubes using x-rays following injection of a contrast medium

*salping*o-oophorectomy surgical removal of the fallopian tube and ovary. May be unilateral or bilateral.

*salping*opexy surgical fixation of the fallopian tube

*salping*opharyngeal muscle pertaining to the muscle that widens the pharynx when eating and the eustachian tube when it is blocked. The latter movement alleviates the earache when descending from high altitudes.

-salpinx fallopian tube; uterine tube

hemato*salpinx* accumulation of blood in the fallopian tube

hydro*salpinx* accumulation of watery fluid in the fallopian tube

pyo*salpinx* accumulation of pus in the fallopian tube

salt An inorganic compound that contains a negative ion of an acid with a positive ion of a base.

sarc/o flesh

*sarc*olemma cell membrane of a muscle cell

*sarc*oma malignant tumor of connective tissue such as cartilage, bone, and muscle

*sarc*omere portion of skeletal muscle that contracts to produce movement

*sarc*oplasm cytoplasm of a muscle cell

saturated fatty acids See **fatty acids**.

scans of nuclear medicine

A diagnostic test in which a radioactive substance is injected, swallowed, or inhaled into the body. A specialized camera, called a gamma camera, detects the substance as it accumulates in the body area being studied.

bone s.: detects bony injury, pathology, and repair. The intra-venously injected radioactive substance is absorbed by bone tissue, following which a gamma camera is used to produce and record an image.

brain s.: demonstrates metabolic and functional processes, as well as brain lesions. Following intravenous injection of a radioactive substance, such as technetium-99m, images are obtained that demonstrate the cerebral blood vessels. In healthy individuals, the blood-brain barrier (BBB) prevents technetium-99m from entering the brain tissues. However, in disease, injury, or other brain pathology, the BBB breaks down allowing technetium-99m to pass through the BBB and be absorbed. The gamma camera can detect the accumula-tion of the radioactive substance, thereby producing and recording an image. Brain images are used for studying men-tal disorders, epilepsy, and degenerative diseases of the brain.

cardiac s.: following injection of a radioactive substance and its uptake by the myocardium, images of the heart are produced as it beats, and the volume of blood pumped by each ventricle can be accurately measured.

gallium s.: radioactive gallium is intravenously injected. A gamma camera is used to detect the areas in which gallium accumulates, producing and recording an image of that area. The uptake of gallium is seen in some tumors and infections.

HIDA scan: following injection of HIDA, a radionuclide, images of the liver and gallbladder, and patency of the biliary tree are studied.

Memory Key: HIDA is an abbreviation for hepatoimino-diacetic.

positron emission tomography (PET): studies meta-bolic activity of a structure. Radioactive particles called *positrons*, released from radioactive substances, are injected into the body, settling in areas such as the heart and brain. The location of the radioactive substance shows up in cross-sectional, color-coded images. Through these colored pictures, metabolic processes of the brain and other structures can be studied. Used to diagnosis schizophrenia, epilepsy, migraine headaches, and strokes.

pulmonary perfusion s.: demonstrates blood flow through the lung. A radioactive substance is injected and flows to the lungs. A gamma camera produces an image of the distribution of blood around the alveoli that highlights the areas that have obstructed blood flow and, therefore, no uptake of the radioactive substance.

pulmonary ventilation s.: demonstrates pulmonary function. Xenon gas is inhaled and the distribution of air within the lungs is demonstrated by the gamma camera.

thyroid s.: demonstrates which part of the gland might be functioning at an accelerated or depressed rate. A radioactive substance, such as technetium-99m, is intravenously injected, settling in the thyroid gland, and an image is produced using a gamma camera.

scaphoid   One of eight carpal bones. See **carpal bones** under **carp/o**.

scapul/o   scapula; shoulder blade

scapula   one of two triangular-shaped bones located bilaterally on the back of the thoracic cage below the shoulders

Memory Key: Compare the spelling of scapul**a**, the noun form, with its adjectival form, scapul**ar**.

scapular   pertaining to the shoulder blade. See Memory Key following above.

scar   A mark left on the skin following healing of a wound, due to the infiltration of connective tissue cells to the site of injury. Also known as *cicatrix*.

-schisis cleft; split; abnormal fissure

cheilo*schisis* congenital splitting of the upper lip. See **cheil/o, cheiloschisis**.

myelo*schisis* splitting of the spinal cord

palato*schisis* congenital splitting of the palate. See **palat/o, palatoschisis**.

rachis*chisis* congenital splitting of the vertebral column. See **spina bifida**.

retino*schisis* splitting of the retina.

Schwann cell   Cells of the myelin sheath that wrap some axons of the peripheral neurons.

sciatic nerve   The longest nerve in the body, extending from the sacral plexus down the back of the thigh.

sciatica   Pain of the sciatic nerve.

scler/o hard

amyotrophic lateral *sclerosis* (ALS) progressive degeneration of the motor neurons of the brain and spinal cord ending in death due to heart and respiratory failure

arterio*sclerosis* hardening of the arteries

scleroderma a chronic systemic disease that causes hardening of the skin and some viscera; the skin feels tough and leathery

sclerotherapy an injection of an irritating substance into a vein causing hardening, obliteration, and scarring of the vein; used to treat varicose veins of the legs, rectum (hemorrhoids), and esophagus

scler/o sclera

sclera white outer coat of the eyeball continuous with the cornea

Memory Key: Compare the spelling of scler**a**, the noun form, with its adjectival form, scler**al**.

scleral pertaining to the sclera. See Memory Key above.

***sclero*conjunctivitis** inflammation of the sclera and
  conjunctiva
***sclero*choroiditis** inflammation of the sclera and choroid
  of the eye

-sclerosis hardening

arterio*sclerosis* hardening of the arteries
athero*sclerosis* type of arteriosclerosis characterized by the
  accumulation of a fatty plaque, called *atheroma*, on the walls
  of the artery
phlebo*sclerosis* hardening of the veins

scoliosis Abnormal lateral curvature of the spine.

-scope instrument used to view

endo*scope* an instrument used to view the inside of a hollow
  organ or cavity. Like a telescope, endoscopes are equipped
  with a light viewing apparatus, and power source; attach-
  ments can include a cutting instrument for removal of tissue,
  and suction accessories. Specific types of endoscopes are
  named after the organ or cavity being examined, such as:
  arthroscope (joint)
  bronchoscope (bronchus)
  gastroscope (stomach)
  laparoscope (abdomen)
  otoscope (ear)
  rectoscope (rectum)
  sigmoidoscope (sigmoid colon)

-scopy process of visual examination
using a scope

endo*scopy* the process of visually examining the inside of a
  hollow organ or cavity with an endoscope. Specific types of
  endoscopies are named after the organ or cavity being
  viewed. For example:
  arthroscopy (joint)
  bronchoscopy (bronchus)
  colonoscopy (colon)

esophagoscopy (esophagus)

laparoscopy (abdomen)

ophthalmoscopy (eye)

scrotum External sac of the male reproductive system containing the testicles.

sebaceous gland See **gland**.

seb/o sebum

seborrhea excessive secretion of sebum

sebum oily substance secreted by the sebaceous glands, making skin and hair soft and pliable

secretin A hormone secreted by the small intestine that has a stimulating effect on many digestive system functions.

secretion A substance that is produced and secreted by glands.

sect/o to cut

bisection cutting into two parts

dissection separation of body parts for studying

Memory Key 1: dis- means "apart."

Memory Key 2: Note that dissection is spelled with a double **s**, while bisection and transection have one **s**.

section process of cutting; the cutting away of tissue from an organ for microscopic or macroscopic examination; the sectioning or division of tissue

transection to cut across

secundi second

secundigravida a woman pregnant for the second time. Written gravida II or GII.

secundipara a woman who has twice given birth (500 g or 20 weeks gestation), regardless of whether it was alive or dead. Written para II or PII.

seizure
A single episode of epilepsy characterized by attacks of altered cerebral functions and muscle contractions (convulsions) due to uncoordinated and disorganized electrical impulses of the brain. Types include:

generalized s.: involves widespread areas of the brain. Examples include:

absence (petit mal) s.: brief attacks lasting 1 to 30 seconds. The seizure is manifested by blank stares and eye disturbances. If there is a loss of consciousness, it is so brief, a matter of seconds, that it goes unnoticed.

tonic-clonic (grand mal) s.: alternating tonic contractions (prolonged contraction with no muscle relaxation) and clonic contractions (alternating muscular contractions and relaxation)

partial s.: a seizure that originates in a localized or specific area of the brain.

selective semipermeable membrane
The cell membrane that regulates the movement of substances into and out of the cell.

sella turcica
Saddle-shape depression in the sphenoid bone; contains the pituitary gland.

semen
Thick, sticky fluid that is ejaculated from the male reproductive tract; formed from sperm and other substances secreted from reproductive glands.

semi- half

semicircular canals part of the bony labyrinth of the inner ear that maintains balance; contains perilymph; shaped as half circles

semicircular ducts part of the membranous labyrinth of the inner ear that maintains balance; contains endolymph; shaped as half circles

***semi*comatose** state of unconsciousness from which the patient may be aroused. In this case, **semi-** means "almost, but not quite" as "not quite in a coma, but almost."

***semi*lunar cartilage** see **meniscus**

***semi*lunar valves** see **valve**

seminal vesicle
One of two structures of the male reproductive system that secretes a thick, alkaline fluid into the ejaculatory duct. (See Appendix F, Figure 17.)

seminiferous tubules
Tightly coiled tubes in the testicles that produce sperm.

sensation
The stimulation of afferent (sensory) receptors that results in a feeling or awareness of conditions internal and external to the body.

sense
Awareness by the central nervous system of conditions external and internal to the body.

sensory neuron
Sensory (afferent) neurons transmit impulses to the brain and spinal cord.

sensory receptor
Sensory nerve endings that receive internal and external stimuli.

sensory system
Afferent system. See **system**.

sepsis
Noun indicating a toxic state resulting from the infection of blood and tissues by microorganisms.

-sepsis, -septic infection
anti*sepsis* the prevention of an infection by impeding the growth of the causative microorganism

a*septic* free from infectious material

septum
A wall dividing two cavities. Examples include:
atrial s.: divides the atria of the heart into right and left portions.

nasal s.: divides the nasal cavity into right and left halves.

ventricular s.: divides the ventricles of the heart into right and left portions.

ser/o serum

serous fluid watery fluid secreted by serous membrane

serous membrane a membrane composed of epithelial tissue found in cavities that do not lead to the exterior; specifically the peritoneal, pleural, and pericardial cavities. Also known as *serosa*. Types of serous membrane include:

parietal m.: serous membrane that **lines** cavities that do not lead to the exterior.

visceral m.: serous membrane that **covers** organs in cavities that do not lead to the exterior.

serum (1) Plasma minus the clotting elements such as fibrinogen and prothrombin. (2) watery fluid moistening the surfaces of serous membranes.

serosa Serous membrane See **ser/o, serous membrane**.

serotonin (1) A vasoconstrictor found in many body organs. (2) A neurotransmitter secreted by some neurons.

Sertoli cells Cells found in seminiferous tubules.

sesamoid bone A small oval-shaped bone embedded in a tendon lying over a joint, such as the kneecap; a sesamoid bone does not articulate with another bone.

sex chromosome The gender-determining chromosome; in females it is XX and in males it is XY.

sex-linked gene See **X-linked gene**.

sex-linked trait See **X-linked trait**.

sexually transmitted disease A variety of diseases transmitted by sexual contact, including aids, syphilis, gonorrhea, genital herpes, and Chlamydia; venereal disease.

shaft The diaphysis of a long bone; the long, slender portion of a long bone between the bulbous ends.

shingles An infection of cranial and spinal nerves. See **herpes zoster**.

shock A sudden reduction in blood pressure. Due to vasodilation, there is effusion of fluid out of the blood vessel and into the surrounding tissues, blood pressure is reduced, and blood flow to organs becomes inadequate.

    anaphylactic s.: shock due to acute hypersensitivity to an antigen that results in symptoms that include hives, pruritus, and life-threatening dyspnea and shock.

    cardiogenic s.: shock due to the failure of the heart to pump adequate quantities of blood

    hemorrhagic s.: shock due to the loss of large amounts of blood

    hypovolemic s.: shock due to a decrease in blood volume

    neurogenic s.: shock due to vasodilation caused by trauma to the central nervous system

sialaden/o salivary gland

*sialaden*itis inflammation of the salivary gland

sial/o saliva

*sial*olith stone in the salivary gland or duct

sickle-cell anemia See **anemia**.

sigmoid/o sigmoid colon

sigmoid colon s-shaped portion of the colon between the descending colon and rectum. (See Appendix F, Figure 6.)

Memory Key: Sigmoid refers to the Greek letter sigma (Σ), which is equal to the letter "s" in our alphabet.

sigmoidoscopy process of viewing the sigmoid colon

sign
Objective symptoms of disease that the physician notices, such as paralysis or erythema. Compare with **symptom**.

silicosis
An accumulation of silica dust in the lung. See **pneum/o, pneumoconiosis**.

simple fracture
A fracture in which the bone does not break the skin; closed fracture. (See Appendix F, Figure 20.)

simple squamous epithelium
Epithelial tissue composed of flat, platelike cells arranged in a single layer.

sinoatrial node
Part of the independent electrical system of the heart. See **conduction system**. (See Appendix F, Figure 3.)

sinus
(1) Cavity or space within a structure. For example, the **paranasal sinuses** are cavities within the skull bones, located near the nose. There are four paranasal sinuses: **frontal, maxillary, sphenoidal, and ethmoidal**. (2) An abnormal passageway to allow pus to drain from an abscess.

sinus/o sinus
***sinus*itis** inflammation of the paranasal sinuses
***sinus*otomy** incision into the sinus

skeletal muscle
See **muscle**.

skeletal muscle tissue
Tissue composed of elongated, multinucleated, striated cells making up skeletal muscles.

skeletal system
See **system**.

skin
The organ composed of epithelial tissue, consisting of the dermis and epidermis. (See Appendix F, Figure 22.)

skull The bony structure of the head. See **cranial bones**. (See Appendix F, Figure 19.)

sliding filament theory A theory of muscle contraction in which the myofilaments of a muscle slide past each other rather than shorten.

slipped intervertebral disc See **herniated disc**.

slough Necrotic tissue that is shed from the tissue below; in ulcers necrotic tissue is sloughed off leaving an open sore.

small bowel follow through See **barium studies**.

small bowel series See **barium studies**.

small intestine The portion of the intestine between the stomach and cecum; includes the duodenum, jejunum, and ileum. (See Appendix F, Figure 6.)

smooth muscle Muscle of internal organs that are nonstriated due to the lack of alternating dark and light bands in each muscle fiber.

sodium An alkaline, metallic chemical element; one of the main cations in the body.

sodium-potassium pump See **Na$^+$-K$^+$**.

solute A substance that is dissolved in a liquid.

solution Dissolved substances in a liquid.

solvent The liquid in which the solute (substance) will dissolve.

somat/o body

somatic pertaining to the body

somatic cell all undifferentiated cells of the body

somatic nervous system see **system**

somatic reflex reflex action produced by skeletal muscles

somatotrophin hormone secreted by the anterior pituitary gland that stimulates growth in all body cells. Also known as *somatotrophic hormone* or *growth hormone*.

somatomedin A hormone secreted from the liver that stimulates growth of all body cells.

-some body

chromosome structure containing DNA in the nucleus of the cell

lysosome cytoplasmic organelle. See **lys/o**.

son/o sound

sonogram record of an organ or structure obtained by ultrasound

sonolucent structures that allow the passage of ultrasound waves without giving off echoes (reflecting them back to their source).

-spadias opening; split

epispadias congenital opening of the meatus on the dorsum (top side) of the penis

hypospadias congenital opening of the meatus on the ventral (underside) of the penis

-spasm sudden, involuntary muscle contraction

blepharospasm sudden, involuntary contraction of the eyelid muscle

enterospasm sudden, involuntary contraction of the intestinal muscles

esophagospasm sudden, involuntary contraction of the esophageal muscles

gastro*spasm* sudden, involuntary contraction of the stomach muscles

myo*spasm* sudden, involuntary muscle contraction

spatial summation
A process in which postsynaptic potentials generated in different regions of a postsynaptic cell may work together to trigger a signal.

special senses
Hearing, smell, sight, equilibrium, touch, and taste

spermat/o sperm

***spermatic* cord** a tough, fibrous cord extending from the inguinal ring to the testicles; composed of a group of structures including the vas deferens, as well as the arteries, veins, and nerves leading to the testicles

spermatocyte an immature sperm cell

spermatogenesis formation of sperm

spermatozoa mature sperm cells produced by the testicles to fertilize an ovum. Singular is spermatozoon.

spermicide
Agent that kills sperm.

sphenoid bone
One of the bones of the skull.

Memory Key: Sphen/o means "wedge," because it occurred to early anatomists that the sphenoid bone was wedged between the temporal bones.

sphincter
A circular muscle that allows the passage of material when the muscle is relaxed and restricts the passage of material when the muscle closes. Examples include:

anal s.: muscle that closes the anus

cardiac s.: located at the distal end of the esophagus as it enters the stomach. Opens to allow passage of food into the stomach and closes to prevent stomach contents from re-entering the esophagus. Also known as *lower esophageal sphincter*.

lower esophageal s.: see **cardiac sphincter**.

pharyngoesophageal s.: located between the pharynx and esophagus; opens at the approach of food and closes at other times to prevent air from entering the stomach. Also known as *upper esophageal sphincter.*

pyloric s.: located at the distal end of the stomach; permits the passage of food from the stomach to the duodenum.

s. of Oddi: located in the common bile duct; opens to release bile and pancreatic juices into the duodenum.

upper esophageal s.: see **pharyngoesophageal sphincter** above.

sphygmomanometer
The instrument that measures blood pressure.

spina bifida
The congenital splitting of the vertebral column. May result in herniation of the meninges as well as the spinal cord, resulting in a multitude of complications depending upon the severity of the hernia and its effect on the transmission of electrical impulses through the spinal cord. Also known as *rachischisis.*

spin/o backbone; spinal column; vertebral column; spine

*spin*al **cavity** area of the dorsal cavity containing the spinal cord. Also known as *vertebral cavity.*

*spin*al **column** bony structure protecting the spinal cord. Includes 33 vertebrae: 7 cervical, 12 thoracic, 5 lumbar, 1 sacrum (5 fused bones), and 1 coccyx (4 fused bones). Extends from the head to the pelvis. Also known as the *vertebral column, backbone,* or *spine.* (See Appendix F, Figure 21.)

*spin*al **cord** nervous tissue in the spinal cavity extending from the foramen magnum at the base of the skull, to between the first and third lumbar vertebra

*spin*al **nerve** a group of nerve cell fibers extending from the spinal cord that carry electrical impulses to and from it

spinal tap removal of cerebrospinal fluid from the subarachnoid space. See **lumb/o, lumbar puncture**.

spine see **spinal column** above

spiral fracture
A fracture line that curves around the bone. (See Appendix F, Figure 20.)

spir/o breathing

Memory Key: Many English words use spir/o as a root, such as *aspir*e (breathe toward), *inspir*e (breathe into), ex**pir**e (to breath out).

aspirate to withdraw fluid, air, or tissue from a cavity

spirometer instrument used to measure air flow and volume into and out of the lungs

spirometry process of measuring air flow and volume into and out of the lungs

spleen
The organ located in the left hypochondrium near the stomach; produces red blood cells, stores blood, removes old blood cells, aids in B-lymphocyte multiplication, and contains many phagocytes. (See Appendix F, Figure 8.)

splen/o spleen

Memory Key: Notice that the root **splen/o** has one **e** and the English word *spleen* has two.

splenectomy surgical removal of the spleen

splenomegaly enlarged spleen

splenorrhagia bleeding from the spleen

splenorrhaphy suturing of the spleen

splenorrhexis ruptured spleen

spondyl/o vertebra

spondylitis inflamed vertebra

spondylopathy disease of the vertebra

spondylosis abnormal condition of the vertebra characterized by immobility of the vertebral joints

spongy bone Bone that looks like a sponge, having many spaces; found in the epiphyses of bones. Also known as *cancellous bone*.

sprain An injury to a joint involving the stretching and tearing of ligaments and tendons. Compair with **strain**.

squamosal suture An immovable joint of the skull. See **suture** definition (3).

squamous Used to describe structures that are scale-like, plate-like, and flat, as in squamous cells that are flat epithelial cells found in the skin and mucous membrane.

squamous cell carcinoma A localized malignant tumor of flat, scale-like cells of epithelial tissue; rarely metastasizes.

staircase phenomenon An effect exhibited by muscle in which each successive contraction in a series is greater than the preceding one. Also known as *treppe*.

staped/o stapes

stapedectomy surgical removal of the stapes and replacement with a prosthesis; this procedure, usually performed for otosclerosis, will restore hearing in most cases.

stapes One of the three ossicles of the middle ear. Also known as the *stirrup*. (See Appendix F, Figure 14.)

staphyl/o bunch of grapes

staphylococcus berry-shaped bacterium growing in clusters, similar to a bunch of grapes; causes pyogenic infections

staphyl/o uvula

staphylorrhaphy suturing of the uvula to correct cleft palate
staphylotomy incision into the uvula. Also known as *uvulotomy*.

Starling's law of the heart
States that the force of contraction of the heart muscle is determined by the length of the fibers; the more fibers stretched by blood filling the ventricles, the more forceful the heartbeat.

-stasis stopping; controlling
hemo*stasis* the stoppage of bleeding or blood flow
homeo*stasis* tendency in an organism to maintain an equilibrium or constant, stable state
meta*stasis* spreading of a malignant tumor from one part of the body to another. **Meta-** means "beyond."

steat/o fat
steat*oma* tumor containing fat; lipoma
steat*orrhea* (1) Discharge of fat in the feces as in pancreatic disease. (2) Increased secretion of sebaceous glands.
cholesteat*oma* see **chol/e**

stem cells
Immature blood cells from which all mature blood cells evolve; found in red bone marrow and lymphatic tissue. Also known as *hemocytoblast*.

-stenosis narrowing; constriction

Memory Key: To remember that **stenosis** means "narrowing," think of a **steno**grapher as a person who writes in shorthand.

angio*stenosis* narrowing of the blood vessels
arterio*stenosis* narrowing of the lumen of an artery often due to the accumulation of fatty plaque on the arterial wall
dacryo*stenosis* narrowing of the lacrimal duct
phlebo*stenosis* narrowing or constriction of a vein
pyloric *stenosis* narrowing of the pyloric sphincter

stere/o solid; having three dimensions
cholesterol see **chol/e**
stere*ognosis* the ability of an individual to identify an object by touch alone. Visualization is not allowed.

stereotaxis a technique employed in brain surgery, using three-dimensional coordinates to precisely locate functional areas of the brain

sterile (1) Free of bacteria or other microorganisms. (2) Unable to produce offspring.

sterilization (1) Process by which all the microorganisms are destroyed in a substance. (2) Operative procedure that renders a person incapable of producing offspring, as in a vasectomy, salpingectomy, tubal ligation, or castration.

stern/o sternum; breastbone

sternal pertaining to the breastbone

Memory Key: Compare the spelling of stern**al**, the adjectival form, with its noun form, stern**um**.

sternoclavicular pertaining to the sternum and collarbone
sternum breastbone; narrow, flat bone in the middle of the chest. See Memory Key above. (See Appendix F, Figure 19.)

steroid An organic compound. Includes D vitamins, bile acids, and certain hormones, such as corticosteroids.

stethoscope An instrument used to listen to bodily sounds as in the lungs and heart.

-sthenia strength

asthenia without strength
myasthenia muscular weakness

stimulus Change in the external or internal environment that can evoke a response.

ST interval Part of the electrocardiogram that indicates the period of time between ventricular contractions.

stoma Surgical creation of a new, artificial opening in the viscera.

stomach An organ of the digestive system located in the left upper quadrant of the abdomen between the esophagus and small intestine.

stomat/o mouth

stomatitis inflammation of the mouth

-stomy new opening

Memory Key: Do not confuse **-stomy** meaning "new opening" with **-tomy** meaning "to cut."

colocolostomy creation of a new opening between two segments of the colon; anastomosis between two segments of the colon. See **ana-, anastomosis**.

colostomy creation of a new opening between the colon and abdominal wall

gastrojejunostomy new opening between the stomach and jejunum; anastomosis between the stomach and jejunum. See **ana-, anastomosis**.

tracheostomy creation of a new opening in the trachea through which a patient can breathe; may be temporary or permanent

stool See **feces**.

strabismus Abnormal deviation of the eyes; cross-eye. See **-tropia**.

strain Over-stretching of muscle usually due to over-exercise or overuse. Compare with **sprain**.

stratified Appearing in layers.

Memory Key: Do not confuse **stratified**, meaning "arranged in layers," with **striated** meaning "striped."

stratified epithelium Epithelial tissue composed of epithelial cells that are arranged in layers.

stratified squamous epithelium Epithelial tissue composed of flat, platelike cells arranged in layers.

stratum Flat structure, particularly those that occur in layers. Used in naming many anatomical structures. Following are the edidermal strata:

s. basale: the deepest epidermal layer responsible for regeneration. The stratum spinosum and basale are often collectively called the *stratum germinativum*.

s. corneum: outermost layer of epidermis

s. granulosum: epidermal cells die in this layer.

s. lucidum: consists of dead or dying epidermal cells; found only in the soles of the feet and the palms of the hand

s. spinosum: cells actively grow in this layer. Also known as the *prickle-cell layer*.

streptococcus A berry-shaped bacterium growing in twisted chains; causes pyogenic infections.

stress fracture A slight disruption of bone due to continuous impacts, such as running or jumping.

stressor An unpleasant or threatening occurrence.

stretch receptor Sensory receptors in a muscle that detect muscle stretching.

stretch reflex A spinal cord reflex in which a muscle that is stretched will contract.

stria A line or narrow band. Plural is *striae*

striated Striped; characterized by striae.

Memory Key: Do not confuse **striated**, meaning "striped" with **stratified**, meaning "appearing in layers."

striated involuntary muscle Cardiac muscle. See **muscle, cardiac**.

striated muscle Muscle tissue that appears striped or striated due to the alternating pattern of dark and light bands in each muscle fiber. Skeletal and cardiac muscle are examples of striated muscle.

striated voluntary muscle Skeletal muscle. See **muscle, skeletal**.

stricture A narrowing or constriction of the lumen of a tube, duct, or hollow organ, such as an artery or ureter.

stroke See **cerebr/o, cerebrovascular accident**.

stroke volume The quantity of blood a ventricle ejects per beat.

sty, stye Inflammation of one or more sebaceous glands of the eyelid; hordeolum.

sub- under; below

*sub*acute describes a disease as not quite acute, but not chronic either; somewhere in between acute and chronic. Compare with **acute** and **chronic**.

*sub*arachnoid space space below the arachnoid membrane that is located around the brain and spinal cord; contains cerebrospinal fluid

*sub*clavian below the clavicle or collarbone, as the subclavian artery

*sub*costal pertaining to under the ribs

*sub*cutaneous pertaining to under the skin. Also known as *hypodermic*.

Memory Key: The prefixes **sub-** and **hypo-** must be retained with the roots **cutane/o** and **derm/o** respectively;

therefore, it is always *subcutaneous* and *hypodermic* but never *hypocutaneous* or *subdermic*.

subdural space space between the dura mater and arachnoid membrane of the meninges

sublingual glands salivary glands located under the tongue

subluxation partial or incomplete dislocation of a joint. *Luxation* means "to dislocate."

submandibular glands salivary glands located under the lower jaw

submucosa layer of connective tissue under the mucous membrane. In the digestive tract, it contains lymph vessels, blood vessels, and neurons.

subscapular under the scapula

substantia nigra Gray matter deep in the cerebrum; degeneration of the substantia nigra occurs in Parkinson's disease.

substrate The substance acted upon by enzymes.

sucrase An enzyme secreted by the small intestine to break down sucrose into glucose and fructose.

sucrose A disaccharide broken down into glucose and fructose by the action of sucrase.

sudoriferous gland Sweat gland; see **gland**.

sulcus A groove or depression on the surface of a structure, such as the brain.

summation The process in which a number of stimuli are added together producing a reaction in a nerve or muscle cell.

superficial Positioned near the surface.

superficial reflex See **reflex**.

super/o above

superior above; toward the head

supination (1) The act of turning the palms forward or
up. (2) The act of lying face up on the back. Compare with
pronation.

Memory Key: To remember that the face and palms are
facing up, note that the word s**up**ination contains the word **up.**

supine (1) Palms are turned forward or up. (2) Lying on
the back, face up. A common phrase on an operative report is,
"with the patient in the supine position." See Memory Key
under **supination**.

suppressor T-lymphocyte A blood cell that
regulates the immune system by switching off other cells of
immunity.

supra- above

*supra**ciliary*** pertaining to eyebrows

Memory Key: The **cilia** referred to in this term are the
eyelashes; hence, above the eyelashes are the eyebrows.

*supra**patellar*** above the knee
*supra**renal*** above the kidney

surfactant A natural substance produced by the lungs
to keep the alveoli inflated.

suspension A mixture in which particles are dispersed
but not dissolved in a medium, such as a liquid.

suspensory ligaments Bands of fibrous
connective tissue holding the uterus or the lens of the eye in
place. (See Appendix F, Figures 16 and 15.)

sutural bone Tiny bones located in the joint of the
skull; also called *wormian bones*.

suture (1) As a noun, **suture** refers to the material used to sew up a wound or tie a blood vessel. (2) As a verb, **suture** is the act of sewing up a wound or tying a blood vessel. (3) A type of joint between two immovable surfaces, as in the skull. Types include the **coronal** suture joining the frontal and parietal bones, **lambdoidal** suture joining the occipital and parietal bones, **squamosal** suture uniting the temporal and parietal bones, and the **sagittal** suture joining the parietal bones.

Memory Key: Sagittal comes from the Latin word meaning "arrow"; the position of the arrow as it penetrates the skull from front to back would lie along the sagittal suture.

swayback See **lordosis**.

sweat gland See **gland, sudoriferous**.

sym-, syn- together; with; joined; in connection with

symblepharon adhesion (sticking) of the eyelid to the eyeball

symmetry like parts on opposite side of the body are similar in form, size, and position

symphysis pubis union between the pubic bones at the midline by fibrocartilage; bony prominence under the pubic hair. (See Appendix F, Figure 19.)

synarthrosis an immovable joint in which the bones are united by fibrous tissue, as in the skull; a suture line

synchondrosis a type of immovable joint in which the bones are united by cartilage; usually temporary, as the cartilage becomes ossified

syndesmosis a type of immovable joint in which the bones are united by ligaments

syndrome signs and symptoms occurring (running) together and indicating a particular condition or disease

synergist a muscle that assists another muscle in moving a body part. For example, the adductor muscles of the thigh work together to move the leg. **Erg** means "work."

synthesis the combining of smaller elements to create a more complex substance such as the building up of protein from simpler amino acids. **The/o** means "to place."

sympathetic nervous system See **system**.

symptom Any subjective indication of disease that the patient notices, such as stomach ache, ringing in the ears, muscle soreness. Compare with **sign**.

synapse The space between one neuron and another, or between a neuron and a muscle cell through which a nerve impulse is transmitted.

synaptic cleft A small, fluid-filled space between two neurons, or between a motor neuron and a muscle into which neurotransmitters are released.

synaptic knob The end of an axon from which neurotransmitters are released. Also known as *axon terminal*.

synaptic vesicle A small sac at the end of an axon that contains the neurotransmitter.

syncope Fainting.

synechia Adhesions of body parts, particularly the iris to lens and cornea. Plural is synechiae.

synovi/o synovial fluid; synovial membrane

synovia a thick, colorless fluid that lubricates joints, bursae, and tendon sheaths. Also known as *synovial fluid*.

Memory Key: Synovia resembles the white of an egg, hence **syn-** meaning "in connection with" + **ov/o** meaning "egg."

synovial cavity space between two bones in a freely move-able joint

synovial fluid see **synovi/o, synovia**

synovial joint a freely movable joint, such as the knee or shoulder joints

synovial membrane a thin layer of tissue lining a joint cavity and secreting synovial fluid

syphilis
A sexually transmitted disease caused by the microorganism *Treponema pallidum.*

system
An organized grouping of associated structures working together to produce certain functions. Included are:

afferent s.: branch of the peripheral nervous system that carries electrical impulses to the brain and spinal cord. Also known as *sensory system.*

autonomic nervous s.: part of the nervous system regulating the activity of glands and involuntary muscles; includes the sympathetic and parasympathetic systems

blood s.: anatomy and physiology of blood cells and blood formation

cardiovascular s.: the heart and blood vessels through which blood is pumped to body tissues. (See Appendix F, Figures 1, 2, and 4.)

circulatory s.: refers to the vessels carrying blood throughout the body. (See Appendix F, Figures 1 and 2.)

digestive s.: organs involved in the ingestion, digestion, and absorption of food, and the elimination of waste. (See Appendix F, Figure 6.)

efferent s.: branch of the peripheral nervous system that carries electrical impulses away from the brain and spinal cord to the glands and muscles. Also known as *motor system.*

endocrine s.: glands and other structures that secrete hormones into the blood stream. (See Appendix F, Figure 7.)

immune s.: system of cells and molecules dedicated to the body's defense against disease.

integumentary s.: the skin and its accessory organs; *integument* means "covering." (See Appendix F, Figure 22.)

lymphatic s.: a system adjacent to the circulatory system consisting of lymph vessels, lymph nodes, a fluid called lymph, the thymus gland, spleen, tonsils, and Peyer's patches. (See Appendix F, Figure 8.)

muscular s.: all the muscles of the body. (See Appendix F, Figures 9 and 10.)

motor s.: see **efferent system**

nervous s.: system that regulates the body's response to external and internal changes in the environment; consists of the brain, spinal cord, peripheral nerves, and cranial nerves. (See Appendix F, Figures 11, 12, and 13.)

organs of special sense: organs that register sound, sight, taste, smell, and touch. (See Appendix F, Figures 14 and 15.)

parasympathetic nervous s.: part of the autonomic nervous system in which the nerves originate in the cranial and sacral areas and end in involuntary muscles and glands. The nerve impulses are dominant during rest.

peripheral nervous s.: portion of the autonomic nervous system outside the brain and spinal cord. Includes the nerves and ganglia.

reproductive s.: the male and female organ system responsible for the production of gametes, ensures fertilization, and in women, houses the developing young. (See Appendix F, Figures 16 and 17.)

respiratory s.: responsible for moving air into and out of the lungs allowing for the exchange of oxygen and carbon dioxide between the air and blood. (See Appendix F, Figure 18.)

reticuloendothelial s.: refers to cells located at various sites throughout the body that have the capability to phagocytose unwanted material. Cells are located in the liver, spleen, bone marrow, and lymphatic tissue.

sensory s.: see *afferent system* above

skeletal s.: all the bones in the body plus the joints. (See Appendix F, Figures 19 and 21.)

somatic nervous s.: portion of the peripheral nervous system transmitting impulses to and from the skin, skeletal muscles, bones, joints, ligaments, eyes, and ears.

sympathetic nervous s.: Part of the autonomic nervous system in which the nerves originate in the thoracic and lumbar areas and end in involuntary muscles or glands. The nerve impulses prepare the body for flight or fight.

urinary s.: organs responsible for the production and excretion of urine. (See Appendix F, Figure 23.)

systemic Pertaining to the body as a whole.

systemic circulation The movement of oxygenated blood from the left ventricle of the heart to body tissues and the return of deoxygenated blood from the tissues to the right atrium.

systemic infection An infection that has spread throughout the body from its original site.

systemic lupus erythematosus (SLE)
A chronic inflammatory disease of connective tissue that affects the skin, joints, nervous system, kidneys, and mucous membranes.

systole Contraction of the myocardium during the cardiac cycle. In **atrial systole**, the atria contracts, pumping blood into the ventricles; in **ventricular systole**, the ventricles contract, pumping blood into the arteries. Compare with **diastole**.

systolic pressure See **blood pressure**.

tachy- fast
tachycardia fast heart beat
tachypnea fast breathing

taenia coli The flat, longitudinal muscle layer extending the length of the large intestine.

talipes A congenital deformity of the foot; clubfoot.

Memory Key: Talipes is Latin for *clubfoot*, formed from **talus** meaning "ankle" and **ped/o** meaning "foot." With this type of deformity, the ankle joint is twisted out of position.

talus One of seven bones of the ankle. See **tarsal bones**.

target cell A cell that is affected by a particular chemical.

target organ An organ that is affected by a specific hormone or drug.

tarsal bones A group of seven bones making up the ankle. (See Appendix F, Figure 19.) Included are the talus, navicular, cuboid, calcaneus, first cuneiform, second cuneiform, and third cuneiform. **Tarsus** is the noun form.

tarsal gland See **gland, meibomian**.

taste buds Cells of the tongue located in projections called *papillae*, capable of distinguishing four primary tastes: sweet, sour, salt, and bitter. Types of papillae include:

    circumvallate p.: circular projections at the back of the tongue responding to bitter stimuli

    filiform p.: rough surfaces at the front of the tongue that aid in licking

    fungiform p.: rounded projections in the middle and anterior of the tongue, responding to sweet, sour, and salt stimuli

-taxis, tax/o order; arrangement; motion toward or away from

ataxia lack of muscle coordination

chemotaxis the migration of a cell or organism in response to a chemical stimulus. For example, as part of the body's defense mechanism to inflammation, leukocytes migrate to the site of injury in response to chemicals released from bacteria, viruses, or injured tissues.

stereotaxis a technique used in brain surgery to precisely locate functional areas of the brain.

T-cell See **T-lymphocyte**.

tears Watery secretion of the lacrimal glands that constantly washes over the eyes keeping them moist.

technetium The most common radioisotope in nuclear medicine; used in many scans including lung, bone, kidney, and brain. See **radioisotope**.

teeth The bony projections in the upper and lower jaws that function in chewing.

tele- far away; at a distance

tel*e*metry the process by which measurements are recorded at a distance from the subject; the signals are usually transmitted by radio waves. For example, a Holter monitor, attached to the patient's belt with leads attached to the chest, records the action of the heart as the patient goes through a normal daily routine.

tel/o end

tel*o*phase fourth and final stage in mitosis in which two daughter cells are formed

tempor/o temples (lateral sides of the head)

tempor*a*l bone cranial bones located on either side of the forehead above the ears. (See Appendix F, Figure 19.)
tempor*a*l lobe lateral sides of the cerebrum. See **lob/o, lobes of cerebrum**. (See Appendix F, Figure 11.)
tempor*o*mandibular joint the union between the temporal bone and lower jaw bone (mandible)

tendin/o, tend/o, ten/o tendon

tendin*i*tis inflamed tendon
tendin*o*us pertaining to the tendon
ten*o*desis surgical fixation of a tendon to a new point or attachment
ten*o*synovitis inflammation of the tendon sheath. See **tendon sheath**.
ten*o*tomy process of cutting a tendon

tendon The tough, fibrous connective tissue that attaches muscle to bone.

tendon sheath The covering of a tendon; lined with synovial membrane, it secretes synovial fluid preventing friction between the tendon and its sheath.

terat/o monster

teratogen an agent that causes developmental abnormalities in the embryo; may be chemical or microbial

teratoma congenital tumor composed of embryonic cells that have developed into different organs such as bone, hair, and teeth; usually seen on the ovaries or testicles; can be benign or malignant

testis The male gonad or testicle; plural is *testes.*

test/o, testicul/o testis; testicle

testectomy excision of a testicle

testicular pertaining to the testicles

testosterone The male sex hormone secreted by the interstitial cells of Leydig for the development of male reproductive organs and secondary sex characteristics.

tetanus (1) Sustained muscle contraction in response to repetitive stimulation; tonic contraction. (2) An infectious disease characterized by severe muscle spasms, caused by the bacterium *Clostridium tetani.*

tetany Intermittent and painful muscle spasms of the extremities due to calcium imbalance.

tetrad A group of four common entities, such as the grouping of four chromosomal elements, that occurs at the beginning of meiosis.

thalam/o thalamus

thalamocortical pertaining to the thalamus and cerebral cortex

thalamus a brain structure located below the cerebrum that functions as a relay center for sensory impulses on their way to the cerebral cortex

thel/o nipple

endo*thel*ium flat, scale-like epithelial tissue that lines internal organs, such as the blood vessels, heart, and lymph vessels. See Memory Key under below.

epi*thel*ium tissue forming the epidermis of the skin and the outer layer of the mucous and serous membranes

Memory Key: Originally, **epithelium** referred to the tissue upon the nipple (**thel/o** means "nipple"). Over time, however, **epithelium** took on a broader meaning, "with reference to the skin," but the root **thel/o** was not changed to represent the more modern definition. To add further confusion, **endothelium** and **mesothelium** were coined with the same root **thel/o** to describe tissue that had nothing to do with the nipple.

meso*thel*ium epithelial tissue that lines the peritoneal, pleural, and pericardial cavities and covers the organs in them. See Memory Key above.

poly*thel*ia more than the usual pair of nipples

***thel*itis** inflammation of the nipple

therm/o heat

thermometer instrument used to measure a patient's temperature

thermoreceptor sensory receptors sensitive to changes in temperature; usually located in the skin

-thermy heat

dia*thermy* heat applied to deep tissues

thorac/o chest

***thorac*entesis** see **thoracocentesis** below

***thorac*ic cage** bony structure surrounding the thorax consisting of sternum, costal cartilage, ribs, and thoracic vertebrae

***thorac*ic cavity** hollow space in the chest containing the heart, lungs, bronchial tubes, trachea, esophagus, and large blood vessels; includes the mediastinal cavity between the lungs

thoracic duct left lymphatic duct extending up the midchest area to the subclavian and internal jugular veins; functions to carry lymph to the bloodstream. (See Appendix F, Figure 8.)

thoracic vertebra spinal bones attached to the ribs. See **vertebra**.

thoracocentesis surgical puncture of the chest wall into the pleural cavity to remove fluid. Also known as *thoracentesis*, *pleurocentesis*, and *pleuracentesis*.

thoracodynia chest pain

thoracolumbar pertaining to the chest and lumbar area of the spine

thoracoplasty surgical reconstruction of the chest

thoracotomy incision of the chest wall

thorax
The chest; area of the body between the diaphragm inferiorly and the neck superiorly. (See Appendix F, Figure 19.)

-thorax chest

hemothorax blood in the pleural cavity

hydrothorax fluid in the pleural cavity

pneumothorax air in the pleural cavity

pyothorax pus in the pleural cavity. Also known as *empyema*.

thromb/o clot

thrombocyte cell responsible for clotting; platelet

thrombocytosis slight increase in the number of thrombocytes

thrombocytopenia deficient number of thrombocytes

thrombolysis destruction of thrombocytes

thrombophlebitis inflammation of the vein with clot formation

thromboplastin substance secreted by the platelets following injury; the third clotting factor; Factor III, necessary for blood clotting

thrombopoiesis production of thrombocytes

thrombosis the presence of a blood clot in a blood vessel. For example, coronary thrombosis is a blood clot in a coronary artery that blocks the blood feeding the heart, causing a myocardial infarction (MI) or heart attack.

thrombus a blood clot

Memory Key: -us is a noun ending meaning "a condition" or "thing."

thym/o, thymos/o thymus gland

thymectomy surgical excision of the thymus gland

thymosin hormone secreted by the thymus gland that is active in the immune system

Memory Key: -in is a noun suffix meaning "chemical compound."

thymus gland See **gland**.

thyr/o shield

Memory Key: Thyr/o is derived from the Greek word for shield. The thyroid resembles a shield, hence its name.

thyroid cartilage the most prominent of the laryngeal cartilages; can be felt in the front of the neck. Also known as the *Adam's apple*.

thyroid gland see **gland**

thyroid hormones substances secreted by the thyroid gland including thyroxin and triiodothyronine that are responsible for the regulation of the metabolic rate, and calcitonin that is responsible for regulating blood calcium

thyroiditis inflammation of the thyroid

thyroid scan diagnostic procedure utilizing a radioactive substance and a gamma camera. See **scan**.

thyroid stimulating hormone (TSH) hormone secreted by the anterior pituitary that in turn regulates the hormonal activities of the thyroid gland. Also known as *thyrotrophic hormone* or *thyrotrophin*.

thyrotomy cutting into the thyroid

thyrotrophic hormone see **thyroid stimulating hormone**

thyroxin (T₄) hormone secreted by the follicular cells of the thyroid gland; functions by increasing cellular metabolism and stimulating normal growth of cells. Also spelled *thyroxin**e***.

tibi/o tibia; shin bone

tibia the large bone of the lower leg; shin bone. (See Appendix F, Figure 19.)

tibial pertaining to the shin bone

tibiofibular pertaining to the tibia and fibula

tidal volume (TV) See **pulmonary function test**.

tinea A fungal infection of the skin; commonly called *ringworm* because of the ringlike shape of the invading infection. Tinea infections are named after the area infected. For example:

t. barbae: (beard)

t. capitis: (scalp)

t. corporis: (body)

t. cruris: (groin; jock itch)

t. pedis: (foot; athlete's foot)

t. unguium: (nail; onychomycosis)

tinnitus Ringing in the ears.

tissue A group of cells with similar structure and function. Four major tissue types are:

connective t.: found in tendons, ligaments, blood, bone, cartilage, fat, and blood cells; functions to support and shape the body structures; attaches organs together and holds them in place.

epithelial t.: covers the internal and external surfaces of the body. The internal surface is called *mucous membrane* and the external surface is called the *skin*; functions include protection, absorption, and secretion.

muscle t.: found in the heart, internal organs, and over bones; function is movement.

    nervous t.: consists of neurons and neuroglia; capable of conducting electrical impulses.

tissue fluid   See **inter-, interstitial fluid**.

T-lymphocyte   A class of lymphocyte that includes helper T-cells, killer T-cells, and suppressor T-cells, all especially important in the cell-mediated immune response.

-tocia   labor

dystocia difficult labor

eutocia normal labor

oxytocia quick, rapid labor

-tome   instrument used to cut

dermatome instrument used to cut skin

osteotome instrument used to cut bone

myotome instrument used to cut muscle

tom/o   to cut

Memory Key: In the words below, the word element **tom/o** is used in reference to the way the x-rays seem to "slice" through body tissues, detailing the structure at various depths.

tomogram a record of a specific layer or "slice" of the body made by tomography

tomograph a special type of instrument that moves the x-ray source in the opposite direction to the film. In this manner, preselected tissue is shown in detail, while blurring or eliminating detail not being studied.

tomography a process by which an x-ray beam rotates around the patient while the film is moved in the opposite direction. In this manner, hundreds of x-ray pictures are taken detailing the structure at various depths while the less important information is either blurred or eliminated.

    computed tomography (CT scan): the tomographic information is computer analyzed and converted into a composite picture of the body part. Common body parts studied in this fashion include the brain, kidney, abdomen, and chest. Also known as *computed axial tomography* (CAT scan).

-tomy cutting; incision

Memory Key: There are many medical words ending in **tomy**, too many to list here; however, **-tomy** preceded by almost any number of anatomical roots means "incision into" that anatomical structure.

colotomy incision into the colon
gastrotomy incision into the stomach
osteotomy incision into the bone
tenotomy incision into the tendon
tracheotomy incision into the trachea

tone, muscle The normal flexibility and firmness of muscles; normal, low-level tension present in healthy muscle tissue due to their continual and partial contraction.

tongue The muscular structure on the floor of the mouth that aids in digestion and swallowing of food.

ton/o tone; tension

atony lack of muscle tone
dystonia abnormal muscle tone often resulting in impaired muscle movements
myotonia abnormal muscle tone characterized by prolonged muscular rigidity following contraction
tonic-clonic seizure see **seizure**
tonic contraction see **contraction**
tonometer instrument used to measure intraocular pressure
tonometry measurement of intraocular pressure used for the diagnosis of glaucoma

tonsil A mass of lymphatic tissue located in the pharynx. Includes:

lingual t.: lie on the base of the tongue.

palatine t.: lie on either side of the pharynx at the back of the mouth. These are the tonsils we normally think of when we use the term *tonsil*.

pharyngeal t.: lie on the roof of the pharynx. Commonly called *adenoids*.

tonsill/o tonsil

Memory Key: Note that the word root **tonsill/o** has two **l**s while the English term tonsil has one **l**.

tonsillar pertaining to the tonsils

tonsillectomy excision of the tonsils

tonsillitis inflammation of the tonsils

tonsillotome instrument used to cut the tonsils

torti- twisted

torticollis continuous contraction of the sternocleidomastoid muscle of the neck. Also known as *wryneck*. Literal translation is "twisted neck."

total lung capacity (TLC) See **pulmonary function test**.

tox/o toxin; poison

Memory Key: The noun suffix **-in** means "chemical compound."

antitoxin a substance that inhibits the effect of the poisonous substance

toxin a substance that is poisonous to the body

endotoxin poisonous substance in bacteria that is released only when the bacteria starts to degenerate

exotoxin poisonous substance secreted by living bacterial cells

trabecula Strands of connective tissue extending from the sides of an organ into its interior, forming a lattice-like network. Examples are found in the epiphyses of long bone, the canal of Schlemm in the eye, and between the arachnoid and pia mater in the brain.

trace elements
Small amounts of elements found in the body for normal functioning.

trache/o trachea; windpipe

trachea cylindrical cartilaginous tube of the respiratory tract extending from the larynx to the bronchial tubes for the passage of air

tracheoesophageal pertaining to the trachea and esophagus

tracheostomy creation of a new opening in the trachea through which a patient can breathe; may be temporary or permanent

tracheotomy incision into the trachea

trachoma
Contagious conjunctivitis caused by *Chlamydia trachomatis*.

tract
(1) Hollow passages or tubes, such as the digestive, respiratory, or reproductive tracts. (2) A bundle of axons in the central nervous system.

trans- across

transcellular fluid part of the extracellular fluid that is secreted by cells. Examples include peritoneal fluid, pleural fluid, pericardial fluid, aqueous humor, vitreous humor, endolymph, and perilymph.

transhepatic pertaining to across the liver

transurethral pertaining to across the urethra as in transurethral resection of the prostate. See **prostat/o, prostatectomy**.

transverse colon portion of the large intestine that extends across the abdominal cavity under the diaphragm from the liver to the spleen

transverse fracture a fracture line that runs at right angles to the axis of the bone

transverse plane see **plane**

***transverse* tubules** invaginations of the plasma membrane in skeletal or cardiac muscle that form transverse tubules, which look like a "T." Transverse tubules serving to spread electrical excitation within a muscle cell leading to contraction. Also known as *T tubules*.

transcription
The process by which messenger RNA is produced from the information in DNA.

transfusion
The injection of whole blood or blood parts into the blood stream.

transient ischemic attacks
Temporary hold back of blood from areas of the brain; "little strokes."

transitional epithelium
A type of epithelium that changes shape from round to flat as the organ changes shape. For example, the epithelium of the urinary bladder will change shape as it stretches to accommodate urinary filling.

translation
In genetics, the production of protein by using the coded information in messenger RNA.

trapezium
One of eight carpal bones. See **carpal bones** under **carp/o**.

trapezoid
One of eight carpal bones. See **carpal bones** under **carp/o**.

trauma
Emotional or physical injury.

tremor
Involuntary shaking, quivering, or trembling. Types include:

intention t.: one that has become evident when there is voluntary movement, such as a shaking hand while reaching for a pen.

resting t.: an existent tremor when the part is at rest.

treppe See **staircase phenomenon**.

tri- three

tricarboxylic acid cycle see **Krebs cycle**

triceps having three heads or divisions

triceps brachii posterior muscle of the upper arm. See **-ceps**. (See Appendix F, Figure 10.)

tricuspid valve right atrioventricular valve. See **valve**.

trigeminal neuralgia severe nerve pain along the 5th cranial nerve, known as the *trigeminal nerve*.

Memory Key: The trigeminal nerve is so named because it has three branches, extending to the eye, maxilla, and mandible.

trigone region of the bladder so named because the two openings from the ureters together with the opening of the urethra form three points of a triangle

triiodothyronine (T₃) secreted by the thyroid gland; functions by increasing cellular metabolism and stimulating normal cellular growth

triquetral one of eight carpal bones. See **carpal bones** under **carp/o**. **Triquetral** means "three corners."

trisomy in genetics, when an extra chromosome appears on a normally diploid cell. In trisomy 21, there is an extra chromosome on pair 21 resulting in Down syndrome.

triglycerides Fats made from carbohydrates and stored in adipose tissue.

trochanter The large projection on the upper femur to which the hip and thigh muscles are attached; the **greater trochanter** is located laterally and the **lesser trochanter** is located medially.

troph/o nourishment

trophic hormones substances that regulate the production and release of other hormones from another gland. For example, the hypothalamus secretes trophic hormones that stimulate the pituitary gland to secrete its own hormones.

trophoblast outermost layer of the embryonic blastocyst; will develop into the chorion and amnion

-trophy nourishment

atrophy wasting away. See Memory Key under **a-, atrophy**.

dystrophy abnormal growth or development

hypertrophy an abnormal increase in the size of an organ due to an increase in the size of cells. Compare with **hyperplasia** under **hyper-**.

-tropia turning

esotropia inward turning of the eyeball; strabismus; cross-eye

exotropia outward turning of the eyeball; strabismus; walleye

hypertropia upward turning of the eyeball; strabismus; cross-eye

hypotropia downward turning of the eyeball; strabismus; cross-eye

-tropion turning

ectropion outward turning of the eyelid

entropion inward turning of the eyelid

tropomyosin A muscle protein that inhibits muscle contraction by obstructing the contact between actin and myosin.

troponin A muscle protein that inhibits muscle contraction unless it combines with calcium, thereby clearing the way for actin and myosin interaction, which results in muscle contraction.

true ribs See **ribs**.

true vocal cords Folds of mucous membrane that produce sounds by vibrating as air moves out of the lungs.

trunk The body, excluding the head and limbs

trypsin A digestive enzyme secreted by the pancreas to break down proteins.

Memory Key: Trypsin is considered an enzyme but does not have the traditional **-ase** ending.

trypsinogen The inactive form of the enzyme trypsin found in pancreatic juice.

T tubules See **trans-, transverse tubules**.

tubal ligation The closure of the lumen of the fallopian tube by tying, electrocautery, or the use of clips; a form of sterilization in women.

tubercle Small, rounded projection on bones for attachment of muscles and tendons. The suffix **-cle** means "small"; **tuber/o** means "bump" or "lump."

tuberculosis (TB) An infectious disease caused by the bacteria *Mycobacterium tuberculosis*; usually affects the lung.

tuberosity A large, rounded projection from many bones onto which muscles and tendons are attached.

tubular reabsorption A step in urine formation in which substances necessary to the body are returned to the blood via reabsorption in the peritubular capillaries.

tubular secretion A step in urine formation in which materials are selectively transferred from the blood into renal filtrate to be excreted in the urine.

tubule A small tube.

tumor A new growth or mass of tissue; can be **benign**, in which the tumor cells are encapsulated, preventing the tumor from spreading or the tumor can be **malignant**, in which tumor cells are likely to spread (metastasize).

tunica covering; coat

tunica **albuginea** a sheath of connective tissue covering a
  part or organ
tunica **albuginea testis** a covering of the testicles under the
  tunica vaginalis
tunica **vaginalis testis** outer covering of the testicles

Memory Key: Do not let the term *vaginalis* confuse you into
thinking that this covering is part of the female reproductive
system. It is not.

turbinate Bones in the nasal cavity; see **nas/o, nasal conchae**.

T waves See **waves**.

tympan/o typmpanic membrane; eardrum

tympanic **membrane** membrane that is stretched across
  the end of the ear canal separating the outer and middle ear.
  Also known as the *eardrum*.
tympanoplasty surgical repair of the eardrum; myringoplasty

tyrosine An amino acid found in many proteins.

ulcer A wearing away and necrosis of the skin or mucous
membrane with sloughing of necrotic tissue, leaving an open
sore. Types include:

  decubitus u.: ulcerative skin lesions caused by constant
  pressure from lying or sitting in one position for too long.
  peptic u.: ulcers that affect the lining of the digestive
  tract (**peptic** means "digestion"); the mucous membrane
  of the stomach and proximal duodenum are most commonly affected.

ulcerative colitis Chronic ulceration of the colon.
See **ulcer**.

-ule Small; little.

lob*ule* a small lobe

tub*ule* a small tube

ven*ule* a small vein

uln/o ulna

ulna the lateral bone of the forearm. (See Appendix F, Figure 19.)

Memory Key: Compare the spelling of uln**a**, the noun form, with its adjective form, uln**ar**.

ulnar pertaining to the ulna. See Memory Key above.

ultra- excess; beyond

***ultra*sonogram** a record or image produced using ultrasound. Also known as an *echogram* or *sonogram*.

***ultra*sonography** see **ultrasound** definition (2)

***ultra*sound** (1) Inaudible sound. (2) Use of high frequency sound waves to record an image of internal structures. This technique allows reflected ultrasounds, called echoes, to form an image of internal structures, such as the brain or fetus. Also known as *ultrasonography* or *echography*.

***ultra*violet (UV)** refers to invisible wavelengths of light above the visible violet light in the color spectrum; used in the treatment of acne and psoriasis. UV light from the sun can cause skin cancer.

-um structure

acetabul*um* hip socket

ili*um* the hip bone; one of the bones of the pelvis

myocardi*um* muscle layer of the heart

sept*um* a wall dividing a cavity; a partition

umbilic/o umbilicus; navel

***umbil**ical* **arteries** two arteries in the umbilical cord that carry deoxygenated blood from the fetus to the placenta

***umbil**ical* **cord** structure that connects the fetus to the placenta; contains two arteries and one vein

***umbil**ical* **hernia** see **hernia**

***umbil**ical* **vein** one vein in the umbilical cord that carries oxygenated blood from the placenta to the fetus

umbilicus the "belly button"; the area in the middle of abdomen that serves for the attachment of the umbilical cord to the fetus

ungu/o nail

peri*ungu*al pertaining to around the fingernail or toenail

Memory Key: Note that the **i** is retained in the prefix even though the root **ungu/o** starts with a vowel.

uni- one; single

***uni**cellular* made up of a single cell. For example, bacterium.

***uni**lateral* pertaining to one side

***uni**polar* **neuron** a neuron with only one process (axon or dendrite) extending from its cell body

universal donor Type O blood; does not have A or B antigens; therefore, can be transfused into all blood types without fear of agglutination.

universal recipient Type AB blood; can receive type A, type B, type AB, and type O blood without fear of agglutination.

unsaturated fatty acids See **fatty acids.**

upper esophageal sphincter The circular muscle at the proximal esophagus. See **sphincter, pharyngoesophageal**.

upper gastrointestinal series See **barium studies**.

upper respiratory infection Infection, often viral, of the upper respiratory tract that includes the nasal cavity and pharynx.

upper respiratory tract Respiratory structures located outside the thoracic cavity, such as the nasal cavity, pharynx, and larynx.

uptake Absorption of a substance, particularly a radiopharmaceutical, into an organ or tissue.

urea End product of protein metabolism; found in the urine.

ureter Two long narrow tubes connecting the kidneys to the bladder. (See Appendix F, Figure 23.)

ureter/o ureter

ureteral pertaining to the ureter

ureterectasis dilatation or stretching of the ureter

ureteroileostomy new opening between the ureter and ileum

ureterolith stone in the ureter

ureterostenosis narrowing of the ureter

ureterostomy new opening between the ureter and abdominal wall; this procedure diverts urine from the ureter to the outside of the body

urethr/o urethra

urethra a tube for the discharge of urine from the bladder to the outside; it is 6 inches long in the male and 1½ inches long in the female. (See Appendix F, Figure 23.)

Memory Key: -a is a noun ending.

urethral orifice see **meatus, urinary meatus**

urethroplasty surgical repair of the urethra

urethrorrhagia bleeding from the urethra

-uria urine; urination

Memory Key: Do not confuse **urea** (end product of protein metabolism) with the suffix **-uria**.

albumin*uria* proteinuria
an*uria* no urine formation. Also known as *urinary suppression*.
bacteri*uria* bacteria in the urine
dys*uria* painful urination
hemat*uria* blood in the urine
noct*uria* frequent urination at night
olig*uria* decreased urination
poly*uria* frequent urination
protein*uria* excessive amounts of protein in the urine; albuminuria
py*uria* pus in the urine

urin/o urine

***urin*alysis** laboratory analysis of urine
***urin*ary bladder** expandable sac located behind the pelvic cavity; acts as a storage vessel in which urine collects before being excreted. (See Appendix F, Figure 23.)
***urin*ary meatus** see **meatus**
***urin*ary retention** buildup of urine in the bladder because of the inability to excrete urine. Compare with **urinary sup-pression** below.
***urin*ary suppression** no urine formation; anuria. Compare with **urinary retention** above.
***urin*ary system** see **system**
***urin*ary tract** the passageway for urine from the kidney through the ureters to the bladder and out through the urethra. (See Appendix F, Figure 23.)
***urin*ary tract infection** infection of the urinary tract, usually the bladder or urethra

ur/o urinary tract; urine

ur*emia* accumulation of waste products in the blood due to loss of kidney function. Also known as *azotemia*.
ur*ogram* record of the urinary tract. Types include:

excretory u.: x-ray of the urinary tract following injection of a contrast medium into a vein. Also known as *intravenous urogram* (IVU) or *intravenous pyelogram* (IVP).

retrograde u.: contrast medium is injected into the ureters through a cystoscope and allowed to flow backward, highlighting the urinary structures. Also known as *retrograde pyelogram*.

urologist specialist in the study of the urinary system in females, and urinary and reproductive systems in males

urology branch of medicine dealing with the diagnosis and treatment of the urinary system in females, and the urinary and reproductive systems in males

urticaria A localized lesion of the skin characterized by the development of wheals and severe itching, usually caused by an allergic reaction. Also known as *hives*.

uter/o uterus

uterine fibroid benign tumor of the uterus. Also known as *uterine myoma, fibroma, leiomyoma, fibromyoma,* or *leiomyoma uteri*.

uterine tubes see **fallopian tubes**

uterosacral pertaining to the uterus and sacrum as in the *uterosacral ligaments* that anchor the uterus to the sacrum

uterovesical pertaining to the uterus and bladder

uterus a hollow organ of the female reproductive system suspended and held in place by ligaments in the pelvic cavity. It is the site in which the fertilized ovum implants and develops. (See Appendix F, Figure 16.)

utricle Membranous sac of the inner ear responsible for balance; contained in the bony vestibule along with the saccule.

uve/o uvea

uvea middle layer of the eye that includes the choroid, ciliary body, and iris

uveitis inflammation of the uvea

uvul/o uvula

uvula a wormlike projection hanging from the soft palate at the back of the mouth

uvulotomy incision into the uvula. Also known as *staphylotomy*.

vacuole A clear space or cavity in the protoplasm of a cell.

vagin/o vagina

vagina a muscular tube extending from the cervix uteri to the outside of the body; serves as the birth canal and receives the penis during sexual intercourse. (See Appendix F, Figure 16.)

vaginitis inflammation of the vagina

vaginomycosis fungal infection of the vagina, an example of which is candidiasis

valgus bent outward

Memory Key: The ending of valg**us** changes depending on the ending of the Latin noun that precedes it.

coxa *valga* outward displacement of the hip joint

genu *valgum* knock-kneed; the knees are close to each other, but the ankles are far apart because the lower leg is bent outward

Memory Key: Genu valgum and ***knock-kneed*** appear to contradict each other; however, think of the ankles as bent outward for this example.

hallux *valgus* displacement of the great toe away from the midline toward the other toes

valve A membranous structure that allows the flow of fluid in one direction only.

aortic semilunar v.: see semilunar valve below.

atrioventricular (AV) v.: heart valve located between the atria and ventricle. (See Appendix F, Figure 4.)

left AV v.: heart valve located between the left atrium and ventricle. Also known as the *bicuspid* or *mitral valve*.

right AV v.: heart valve located between the right atrium and ventricle. Also known as the *tricuspid valve*.

bicuspid v.: left atrioventricular valve, mitral valve. (See Appendix F, Figure 4.)

ileocecal v.: valve located between the ileum (last segment of the small intestine) and the cecum (first segment of the large intestine).

mitral v.: left atrioventricular valve; bicuspid valve. (See Appendix F, Figure 4.)

Memory Key: The valve's two flaps resemble a bishop's hat or miter, hence its name, **mitral** valve.

pulmonary semilunar v.: see semilunar valve.

semilunar v.: half-moon shaped valves located in the heart. Includes:

aortic semilunar v.: valve located on the left side of the heart at the entrance to the aorta. (See Appendix F, Figure 4.)

pulmonary semilunar v.: valve located on the right side of the heart at the entrance to the pulmonary artery. (See Appendix F, Figure 4.)

tricuspid v.: right atrioventricular valve

varic/o varicose veins

varicocele dilatation of the testicular veins inside the spermatic cord

varicose veins dilated and twisted veins, usually of the leg

varus bent inward

Memory Key: The ending of var**us** changes depending on
the ending of the Latin noun that precedes it.

coxa *vara* inward turning of the hip joint

genu *varum* bow-legged; the space between the knees is
abnormally increased, and the lower leg bows inward

Memory Key: Genu varum and *bow-legged* appear to
contradict to each other; however, think of the lower legs as
bowed inward for this example.

hallux *varus* the inward turning of the great toe toward the
midline away from the other toes

vascul/o vessel

vascular pertaining to a vessel

vas vessel

vas deferens tubular structure in the male reproductive system that carries sperm from the epididymis to the ejaculatory duct. (See Appendix F, Figure 17.) Also known as the
ductus deferens.

Memory Key: Deferens means "to carry away from."

vasa recta capillaries of the nephron. Vasa is the plural of vas.

vasa vasorum tiny blood vessels in the walls of larger arteries and veins. Vasa is the plural of vas.

vas/o vessel; duct

vasectomy partial or total removal of the vas deferens (duct
that carries sperm) through an incision in the scrotum;
a sterilization procedure in males

vasoconstriction narrowing of a blood vessel lumen

vasodilatation widening of a blood vessel lumen

vasopressin see **antidiuretic hormone**

vasospasm sudden, involuntary contraction of a vessel resulting in a decrease in the diameter of its lumen

vein A blood vessel carrying blood back to the heart. (See Appendix F, Figure 2.)

vena cava The largest vein in the body. Plural is venae cavae. (See Appendix F, Figure 2.)

inferior vena cava: the vein that returns blood from the lower body to the right atrium.

superior vena cava: the vein that returns blood from the upper body to the right atrium.

venereal disease See **sexually transmitted disease**.

ven/o vein

venostasis stoppage of blood flow in a vein

venous thrombosis a blood clot in a vein

venule small vein

ventilation The movement of air into and out of the lungs.

ventilator A machine that delivers air to a patient's lungs by an endotracheal tube and mechanical pump.

ventricle (1) Lower chambers in the heart pumping blood out of the heart. (2) Four small cavities in the brain containing cerebrospinal fluid.

ventricul/o ventricle

ventriculoperitoneal shunt a procedure used in the treatment of hydrocephalus that diverts excess cerebrospinal fluid from the ventricles of the brain to the peritoneum

ventriculostomy creation of a new opening in the ventricles of the brain to treat hydrocephalus

ventr/o toward the front of the body; toward the belly

ventral cavity open space in the front of the body containing the thoracic, mediastinal, abdominal, and pelvic cavities

ventral column see **anter/o, anterior column**

ventral hernia see **hernia, incisional**

ventral horn see **anter/o, anterior horn**

ventral root see **anter/o, anterior root**

ven/o vein

venule small veins leading from the capillaries

vermiform appendix Structure of the digestive system that hangs onto the cecum. (See Appendix F, Figure 6.)

Memory Key: Vermi means "worm;" **-form** means "shape;" **appendix** means "addition" or "hang on to." The vermiform appendix is a worm-shaped organ that hangs onto the cecum.

verruca A wart; a benign, contagious growth of epithelial tissue caused by the human papilloma virus (HPV).

vertebr/o vertebra

vertebra any one of 33 bones making up the spinal column or backbone. (See Appendix F, Figure 21.) The vertebrae are listed below from superior to inferior. They include:

cervical v.: 7 bones located in the neck. Abbreviated C1 to C7.

thoracic v.: 12 bones located in the dorsal chest. Abbreviated T1 to T12. Also known as *dorsal vertebrae*.

lumbar v.: 5 bones located in the lower back between the thoracic vertebrae and sacrum. Abbreviated L1 to L5.

sacrum: 5 fused bones wedged between both hip bones. Abbreviated S1 to S5.

coccyx: 4 fused bones making up the tailbone

vertebral **cavity** see **spinal cavity**
vertebral **column** see **spinal column**

vertigo Dizziness.

very low density lipoprotein (VLDL)
See **lip/o, very low density lipoprotein**

vesic/o sac; bladder

vesicle an elevated lesion of the skin containing serous (watery) or seropurulent (watery and pus-filled) fluid. Also known as a *blister*. If greater than 1 cm in diameter, called a *bulla* or *bleb*. See Memory Key under **vesical** below.
vesical pertaining to the bladder

Memory Key: It is important to observe the context in which ves**icle** and ves**ical** are used; the pronunciations are similar, but the spellings and meanings are different.

vesicosigmoidostomy new opening between the bladder and sigmoid colon; this procedure diverts urine from the bladder into the sigmoid colon
vesicoureteral pertaining to the bladder and ureters
vesicouterine pouch space between the bladder and uterus; cul-de-sac of Douglas

viable Said of a fetus or newborn capable of living outside of the uterus, at least 500 g or 20 weeks gestation.

villus Hair-like structures projecting from the surface of a membrane. Plural is *villi*.

virulent Extremely toxic; said of a disease that is particularly poisonous.

viscer/o internal organs

viscera internal organs
visceral effectors visceral muscles, cardiac muscles, and glands that are stimulated by motor neurons to produce an effect or response

visceral membrane serous membrane that covers the organs in cavities that do not lead to the exterior, i.e., the pericardial, pleural, and peritoneal cavities

visceral muscle musculature of internal organs. See **muscle**.

visceral pericardium serous membrane covering the heart. Also known as the *epicardium*.

visceral peritoneum serous membrane covering the organs in the abdominal cavity

visceral pleura serous membrane covering the lungs

visceromegaly enlargement of internal organs; organomegaly

viscid Thick, sticky substance.

vital lung capacity The volume of air that can be forcefully expelled from the lungs following deepest inhalation.

vitamins A group of organic substances important to the body's growth and metabolism.

vitiligo Lack of skin pigmentation. See **leukoderma**.

vitre/o glassy; glasslike

vitreous humor glasslike fluid in the posterior cavity of the eye between the lens and the retina

vocal cords Two folds of mucous membrane in the larynx.

false vocal cords: upper folds that do not produce sound.
true vocal cords: lower folds that do produce sounds by vibrating as air moves out of the lungs.

voluntary muscle Skeletal muscle that is controlled by will.

volvulus The twisting of one segment of bowel around another.

vomer bone The thin, flat bone forming the lower portion of the nasal septum.

vomiting The expulsion of gastrointestinal contents through the mouth.

Memory Key: Vomiting has only one **t**.

vulv/o vulva

vulva external genitalia of the female including the labia majora, labia minora, mons pubis, clitoris, and Bartholin's glands

wart A benign papilloma. See **verruca**.

wave A fluctuation seen on recordings, such as electrocardiograms (ECG) and electroencephalograms (EEG).

ECG waves include:

P w.: registers the strength of the atrial contraction.

QRS w.: registers ventricular contraction.

T w.: registers the recovery of the ventricles.

EEG waves include:

alpha w.: is typical of the awake person at rest.

beta w.: occurs during increased activity of the nervous system.

delta w.: is typical of deep sleep.

theta w.: occurs in a person under emotional stress.

wave summation Accumulation of repeated stimuli to a muscle resulting in a contraction of increased strength; occurs when the frequency of stimulation is so rapid that the muscle is unable to relax fully between successive contractions causing tension to build up in the muscle.

wheal A skin lesion characterized by a raised, circular, area of skin usually pale in the center, surrounded by a red discoloration. Examples are mosquito bites and hives.

wheeze An abnormal musical sound heard during inspiration or expiration caused by trapped air.

white blood cell Leukocyte; a mature white blood cell.

white matter Material in the brain and spinal cord that is white in color, representing myelinated neurons.

white muscle Lighter-colored muscle tissue composed of muscle fibers that contract quickly (fast-twitch muscle fibers).

Wilms' tumor See **nephroblastoma**.

wisdom tooth The third molar tooth in the adult mouth.

wormian bones Tiny bones located in the joint of the skull. Also called *sutural bones*.

wrist See **carpal bones**.

wryneck Abnormal continuous contraction of the sternocleidomastoid muscle. See **torticollis**.

xanth/o yellow
*xanth*oma (1) A yellow, circular nodule located in the skin and mucous membrane. (2) A tumor containing fat cells.

xen/o strange

xenograft surgical graft of tissue between different species
xenophobia abnormal fear of strangers

xenon 133 (^{133}Xe) A radioisotope used to assess
air flow through the respiratory tract and blood flow in organs
such as the kidney and brain. See **radi/o, radioisotope**.

xer/o dry

xeroderma skin that is dry and rough
xerophthalmia dryness of the eye, specifically the conjunctiva
  and cornea, due to vitamin A deficiency

X chromosome The chromosome that determines
female characteristics.

xiphoid process The most inferior portion of the
sternum, shaped like the tip of a sword. **Xiph/o** means
"sword."

X-linked gene A gene located on the X chromo-
some but not the Y. Also known as *sex-linked gene*.

X-linked trait A trait induced by a gene located on
the X chromosome but not the Y. Also known as *sex-linked
trait*.

x-rays Electromagnetic radiation of very short wavelengths
that can penetrate through the body onto a photographic film
to produce images of the internal structures of the body; used
for diagnosis and treatment.

yeast infection A fungal infection. See **candidiasis**.

yellow bone marrow Fatty tissue found in the adult's medullary cavity of long bones; does not produce blood cells.

yolk sac An embryonic membrane that produces the embryo's first blood cell.

zinc See **minerals**.

zona girdle or belt

zona **fasciculata** thick middle layer of the adrenal cortex
zona **glomerulosa** thin outer layer of the adrenal cortex
zona **pellucida** thick transparent layer around the oocyte
zona **reticularis** inner layer of the adrenal cortex

zygoma The cheekbone; zygomatic bone. (See Appendix F, Figure 19.)

zygomatic arch The arch formed by the union between the zygomatic and temporal bones.

zygote A fertilized ovum

Appendices

Appendix A

FUNDAMENTAL ELEMENTS OF A MEDICAL WORD

Parts of a Medical Word
Suffix: last part of a word
Prefix: first part of a word
Root: main part of a word

Example: periarthritis
  -itis = suffix
  peri- = prefix
  arthr/o = root

Analysis of Medical Words
Identify the suffix, root, and/or prefix in a medical word.

Define the medical word by starting at the suffix, then go to the beginning of the word—it will be either the prefix or root.
  If there is an additional part to be defined, it will be a root.

Example 1:
  Sub/cutane/ous means pertaining to under the skin.
  -ous is the suffix meaning "pertaining to"
  sub- is the prefix meaning "under"
  cutane/o is the root meaning "skin"

Example 2:
  Electro/cardio/gram means record of the electrical activity of the heart
  -gram is the suffix meaning "record"
  electr/o is the root meaning "electric"
  cardi/o is the root meaning "heart"

Combining Vowel

A combining vowel is a vowel, usually **o**, which combines a root and a suffix, as in cardi**o**logy

OR

two roots as in gastr**o**enterology

HOWEVER,

when the suffix starts with a vowel, the **o** is dropped, as in hepatitis.

Example:
hepat/**o** **+** -itis = hepatitis

Combining Form

The combining form is the root plus the combining vowel.

Example:

arthr	+	o	=	**arthr/o**
↓		↓		↓
root		combining vowel		combining form

Notice that the root is separated from the combining vowel by a slash (/). This is the standard way to write the combining form and indicates that sometimes, and sometimes not, the combining vowel is used in forming medical words.

Appendix B

PRONUNCIATION GUIDE

Syllable Vowel Sound	Pronunciation	Example
tion	shun	regurgitation
short a sound	ah	acute
short e sound	eh	hematemesis
short i sound	ih	adipose
long a sound	ay	pain
long e sound	ee	ileitis
long i sound	igh or eye	rhinitis ileitis
long o sound	oh	anorexia
long u sound	you	acute

PLURAL FORMATION

Use the following rules to a form plural word from its singular form:

1. To form the plural of singular words ending in **is**, change the **is** to **es**.

Singular	Plural
Diagnos**is**	Diagnos**es**
Pelv**is**	Pelv**es**
Neuros**is**	Neuros**es**

2. To form the plural of singular words ending in **us**, change **us** to an **i**.

Singular	Plural
Bronch**us**	Bronch**i**
Bacill**us**	Bacill**i**
Calcul**us**	Calcul**i**
Embol**us**	Embol**i**

    There are a few exceptions. For example, the plural of **virus** is **viruses**, and the plural of **sinus** is **sinuses**.

3. The plural of singular words ending in **a** is formed by adding an **e** to the word.

Singular	Plural
Scler**a**	Scler**ae**
Scapul**a**	Scapul**ae**

4. The plural of singular words ending in **um** is formed by changing the **um** to an **a**.

Singular	Plural
Acetabul**um**	Acetabul**a**
Capitul**um**	Capitul**a**
Sept**um**	Sept**a**
Diverticul**um**	Diverticul**a**

5. The plural of singular words ending in **ix** or **ex** is formed by changing the ending to **ices**.

Singular	Plural
Cal**ix**	Cal**ices**
Cerv**ix**	Cerv**ices**
Ind**ex**	Ind**ices**
Var**ix**	Var**ices**

6. The plural of singular words ending in **oma** is formed by adding a **s** or **ta**.

Singular	Plural
Aden**oma**	adenoma**s**; adenoma**ta**
Carcin**oma**	carcinoma**s**; carcinoma**ta**
Fibr**oma**	fibroma**s**; fibroma**ta**

7. The plural of singular words ending in **nx** is formed by changing the **x** to a **g** and adding **es**.

Singular	Plural
Laryn**x**	Laryn**ges**
Phalan**x**	Phalan**ges**

8. The plural of singular words ending in **on** is formed by changing the **on** to an **a** or simply adding **s**.

Singular	Plural
Gangli**on**	gangli**a**; ganglion**s**

9. The plural of singular words ending in **ax** is formed by changing the **ax** to **aces**.

Singular	Plural
Thor**ax**	Thor**aces**

Memory Key: Remember the following rules:

is	$\rightarrow$	es
us	$\rightarrow$	i
a	$\rightarrow$	ae
um	$\rightarrow$	a
ix	$\rightarrow$	ices
oma	$\rightarrow$	omas; omata
nx	$\rightarrow$	nges
on	$\rightarrow$	a or simply add an s
ax	$\rightarrow$	aces

Appendix D

COMMON SUFFIXES

Suffix	Example	Definition
-a (noun suffix)	conjunctiv**a**	membrane lining the eyelid and covering part of the eyeball
-ac (pertaining to)	cardi**ac**	pertaining to the heart
-al (pertaining to)	ren**al**	pertaining to the kidney
-algia (pain)	ceph**algia**	headache
-ar (pertaining to)	tonsill**ar**	pertaining to the tonsils
-ary (pertaining to)	mamm**ary**	pertaining to the breast
-ase (enzyme)	amyl**ase**	an enzyme that breaks down starch
-cele (hernia; protrusion of an organ through a structure that normally contains it)	cysto**cele**	hernia of bladder
-centesis (surgical puncture to remove fluid)	thoraco**centesis**	surgical puncture of the chest wall to remove fluid
-desis (surgical binding; surgical fusion)	arthro**desis**	surgical fusion of a joint
-dynia (pain)	gastro**dynia**	stomach pain
-eal (pertaining to)	pharyng**eal**	pertaining to the pharynx or throat
-ectasis (dilation, dilatation, stretching)	bronchi**ectasis**	dilation of the bronchus

Suffix	Example	Definition
-ectomy (excision, surgical removal)	tonsill**ectomy**	excision of the tonsils
-emesis (vomiting)	hemat**emesis**	vomiting of blood
-emia (blood condition)	an**emia**	lack of red blood cells or hemoglobin in the blood
-er (one who)	practition**er**	one who has obtained the proper requirements to work in a specific field of study
-gram (record; writing)	cardio**gram**	record of the heart's activities
-graph (instrument used to record)	cardio**graph**	instrument used to record the heartbeat
-graphy (process of recording; producing images)	mammo**graphy**	producing images of the breast by using x-rays
-ia (state of; condition)	anorex**ia**	condition characterized by a loss of appetite
-iasis (abnormal condition)	cholecystolith**iasis**	abnormal condition of stones in the gallbladder
-iatry (medical treatment)	psych**iatry**	a branch of medicine dealing with the study and treatment of mental disorders
-ic (pertaining to)	gastr**ic**	pertaining to the stomach

Suffix	Example	Definition
-ician (a specialist)	phys**ician**	a specialist in the study of medicine who has graduated from a recognized school of medicine and is licensed to practice by the appropriate authorities
-in (chemical substance)	ptyal**in**	chemical substance that breaks down starch
-ine (pertaining to)	uter**ine**	pertaining to the uterus
-ion (process)	sect**ion**	process of cutting
-ior (pertaining to)	anter**ior**	pertaining to the front
-ism (condition)	prognath**ism**	protruding jaw
-ist (specialist)	neurolog**ist**	a specialist in the study of the nervous system and its disorders
-itis (inflammation)	arthr**itis**	inflammation of joints
-lysis (destruction; separation; breakdown)	hemo**lysis**	breakdown of blood
-malacia (softening)	osteo**malacia**	softening of bone
-megaly (enlargement)	cardio**megaly**	enlarged heart
-meter (instrument used to measure)	cranio**meter**	instrument used to measure the skull
-metry (process of measuring)	pelvi**metry**	process of measuring the pelvis
-oid (resembling)	muc**oid**	resembling mucus

Suffix	Example	Definition
-oma (tumor mass)	chondr**oma**	tumor of cartilage
-opsy (to view)	bi**opsy**	microscopic examination of a piece of living tissue that has been excised from the body
-or (one who, that which)	organ don**or**	one who donates
-ose (denotes that a chemical is a carbohydrate; pertaining to)	gluc**ose**, sucr**ose**, lact**ose**, malt**ose** adip**ose**	substances that break down carbohydrates in the small intestine; pertaining to fat
-osis (abnormal condition)	nephr**osis**	abnormal condition of kidney
-ous (pertaining to)	ven**ous**	pertaining to a vein
-pathy (disease process)	myo**pathy**	any disease of a muscle
-penia (decrease, deficiency)	leukocyto**penia**	decrease in the number of white blood cells
-pexy (surgical fixation)	nephro**pexy**	surgical fixation of the kidney
-phobia (irrational fear)	acro**phobia**	fear of heights
-plasty (surgical reconstruction; surgical repair)	rhino**plasty**	surgical reconstruction of the nose; a nose job
-plegia (paralysis)	quadri**plegia**	paralysis of all four limbs
-ptosis (drooping; prolapse, sagging)	blepharo**ptosis**	drooping eyelid

Suffix	Example	Definition
-ptysis (spitting)	hemo**ptysis**	spitting up of blood
-rrhage; **-rrhagia** (bursting forth)	hemo**rrhage** gastro**rrhagia**	bursting forth of blood bleeding from the stomach
-rrhaphy (to suture, sew)	spleno**rrhaphy**	suturing of the spleen
-rrhea (flow; discharge)	oto**rrhea**	discharge from the ear
-rrhexis (rupture)	spleno**rrhexis**	ruptured spleen
-sclerosis (hardening)	arterio**sclerosis**	hardening of the arteries
-scope (instrument used to view)	broncho**scope**	instrument used to view the bronchus
-scopy (process of viewing)	broncho**scopy**	process of viewing the bronchus with the aid of an instrument called a scope
-spasm (sudden, involuntary contraction)	blepharo**spasm**	sudden, involuntary contraction of the eyelid
-stasis (stoppage, controlling)	hemo**stasis**	stoppage of blood
-stenosis (narrowing, stricture)	phlebo**stenosis**	narrowing of a vein
-stomy (new opening)	tracheo**stomy**	new opening into the trachea

Suffix	Example	Definition
-tic (pertaining to)	necro**tic**	pertaining to death of tissue
-tome (instrument used to cut)	osteo**tome**	instrument used to cut bone
-tomy (cutting, incision)	osteo**tomy**	cutting into the bone
-tropia (turning)	eso**tropia**	inward turning of the eyeball
-ule (small, little)	ven**ule**	small vein
-um (structure)	pericardi**um**	structure surrounding the heart
-us (condition, thing)	meat**us**	a passage
-y (process)	neuropath**y** nephropath**y**	disease process of a nerve disease process of the kidney

Suffix Review: Suffixes That Have the Same Meaning

Suffix	Meaning
-ac, -al, -ar, -ary, -eal, -ic, -ine, -ior, -ose, -ous, -tic	pertaining to
-algia, -dynia	pain
-er, -or	one who
-ia, ism, us	condition
-ician, -ist	specialist
-ion, -sis, -y	process
-iasis, -osis	abnormal condition

Appendix E

COMMON PREFIXES

Prefix	Example	Definition
ab- (away from)	**ab**duction	process of drawing away from
ad- (toward)	**ad**duction	process of drawing toward
a(n)- (no, not, lack of)	**a**septic **an**emia	free of infectious material lack of red blood cells
ante- (before)	**ante**natal	before birth
anti- (against)	**anti**biotic	drug used to kill harmful bacteria
bi- (two)	**bi**lateral	pertaining to two sides
circum- (around)	**circum**duction	process of drawing a part in a circular motion
contra- (against, opposite)	**contra**lateral	pertaining to the opposite side
de- (lack of, not)	**de**oxygenated	lacking oxygen
di- (two)	**di**saccharide	a carbohydrate containing two monosaccharides
dia- (through)	**dia**meter	measurement from edge to edge of a circle
diplo- (double)	**dipl**opia	double vision
e- (outward, out)	**e**version	turning a part outward

Prefix	Example	Definition
ec- (out, out of)	**ec**topic	out of place
ecto- (outside)	**ecto**genous	produced outside of the body
endo- (within, innermost)	**endo**scope	instrument used to visually examine within a body cavity or organ
epi- (upon, on, above)	**epi**cardium	structure upon the heart
eso- (inward, within)	**eso**tropia	turning inward of the eyeball
ex- (outside, out)	**ex**cision	process of cutting out
exo- (outside, out)	**exo**tropia	turning out of the eyeball
extra- (outside)	**extra**ocular	outside the eyeball
hemi- (half)	**hemi**plegia	paralysis of one side of the body
hyper- (excessive, above)	**hyper**emesis	excessive vomiting
hypo- (below, under, deficient)	**hypo**gastric	below the stomach
in- (in, into)	**in**cision	process of cutting into
in- (not)	**in**digestible	not capable of being digested
infra- below, beneath)	**infra**costal	pertaining to below the ribs
inter- (between)	**inter**cellular	pertaining to between the cells
intra- (within)	**intra**cranial	within the skull

Prefix	Example	Definition
meso- (middle)	**meso**derm	middle layer of embryonic cells
meta- (beyond, change)	**meta**plasia	change in formation
mono- (one)	**mono**plegia	paralysis of one limb
multi- (many)	**multi**form	having many shapes
nulli- (none)	**nulli**para	a woman who has never given birth
ob- (facing toward, at the back of)	**ob**stetrics	branch of medicine dealing with the management of women during pregnancy, childbirth, and postpartum.
oligo- (scanty; few)	**oligo**spermia	decreased number of sperm
para- (beside, near)	**para**nasal	near the nose
per- (through)	**per**cutaneous	through the skin
peri- (around)	**peri**neuritis	inflammation around the nerve
poly- (many)	**poly**adenoma	tumor of many glands
post- (after)	**post**mortem	after death
pre- (before; in front of)	**pre**natal	before birth
pro- (before)	**pro**drome	symptoms occurring before the onset of disease
retro- (back, behind)	**retro**uterine	behind the uterus

Prefix	Example	Definition
quadri- (four)	**quadri**plegia	paralysis of all four limbs
sub- (under, below)	**sub**cutaneous	under the skin
supra- (above)	**supra**renal	above the kidney
tachy- fast)	**tachy**pnea	fast breathing
trans- (across)	**trans**gastric	pertaining to across the stomach
tri- (three)	**tri**cuspid valve	heart valve with three cusps or projections
uni- (one)	**uni**lateral	pertaining to one side

Prefix Review: Prefixes That Have the Same Meaning

Prefix	Meaning
epi-, hyper-, supra-	above
anti-, contra-	against
circum-, peri-	around
dys-, mal-	bad
ante-, pre-, pro-	before
hypo-, infra-, sub-	below
e-, ec, ecto-, ex-, exo- extra-	outside, out
endo-, intra-	within

Prefix Review: Prefixes That Have the Opposite Meaning

Prefix	Meaning
ab- **ad-**	away from toward
ante-, pre-, pro- **post-**	before after
e-, ec, ecto-, ex-, extra- **endo-, in-, intra-**	out in
epi-, hyper-, supra- **hypo-, infra-, sub-**	above below
tachy- **brady-**	fast slow
hyper- **hypo-**	excessive, above deficient, below
macro- **micro-**	large small
ana- **syn-**	apart together, with, joined

Appendix F

ILLUSTRATIONS

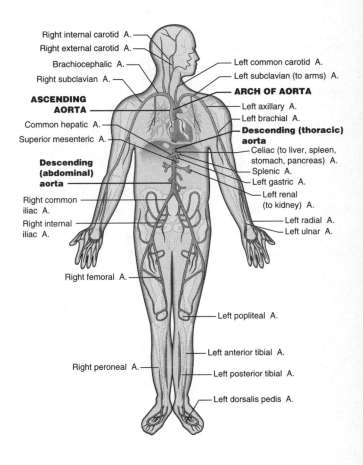

Figure 1
Cardiovascular System (Major Arteries)

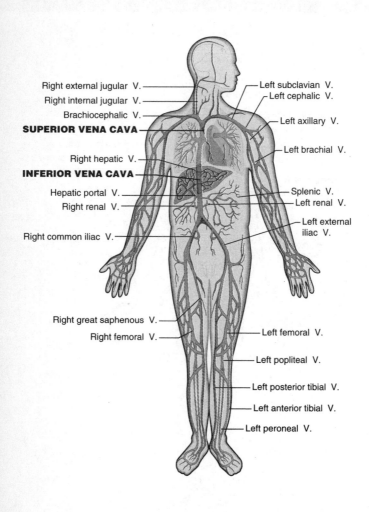

Right external jugular V.
Right internal jugular V.
Brachiocephalic V.
SUPERIOR VENA CAVA
Right hepatic V.
INFERIOR VENA CAVA
Hepatic portal V.
Right renal V.
Right common iliac V.

Left subclavian V.
Left cephalic V.
Left axillary V.
Left brachial V.
Splenic V.
Left renal V.
Left external iliac V.

Right great saphenous V.
Right femoral V.

Left femoral V.
Left popliteal V.
Left posterior tibial V.
Left anterior tibial V.
Left peroneal V.

Figure 2
Cardiovascular System (Major Veins)

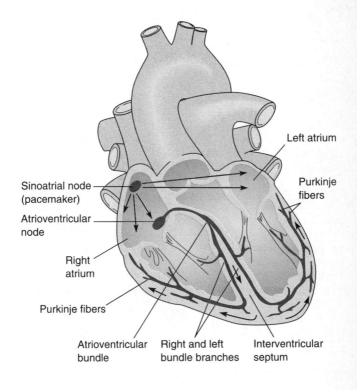

Left atrium

Purkinje
fibers

Sinoatrial node
(pacemaker)

Atrioventricular
node

Right
atrium

Purkinje fibers

Atrioventricular
bundle

Right and left
bundle branches

Interventricular
septum

Figure F-3
Cardiovascular System
(Conduction System)

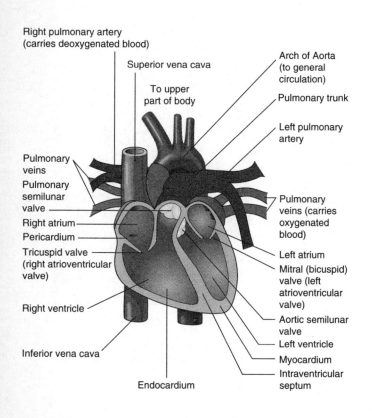

Right pulmonary artery
(carries deoxygenated blood)

Superior vena cava

To upper
part of body

Arch of Aorta
(to general
circulation)

Pulmonary trunk

Left pulmonary
artery

Pulmonary
veins

Pulmonary
semilunar
valve

Right atrium

Pericardium

Tricuspid valve
(right atrioventricular
valve)

Right ventricle

Inferior vena cava

Pulmonary
veins (carries
oxygenated
blood)

Left atrium

Mitral (bicuspid)
valve (left
atrioventricular
valve)

Aortic semilunar
valve

Left ventricle

Myocardium

Intraventricular
septum

Endocardium

Figure 4
Cardiovascular System (Heart)

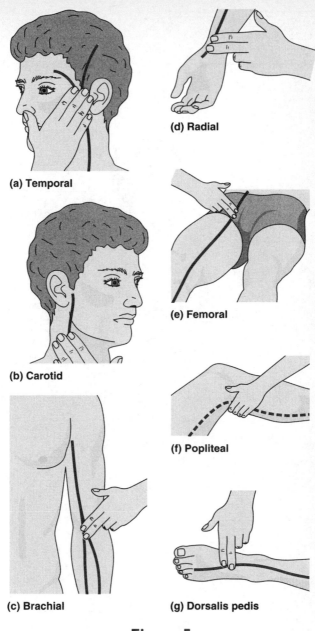

(a) Temporal

(b) Carotid

(c) Brachial

(d) Radial

(e) Femoral

(f) Popliteal

(g) Dorsalis pedis

Figure 5
Cardiovascular System (Pulses)

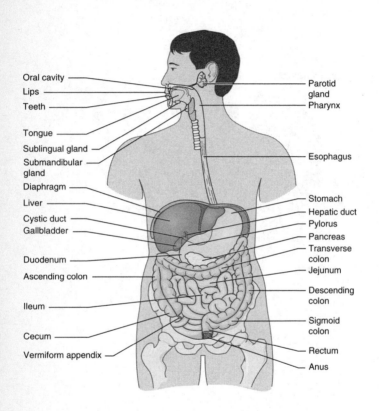

Oral cavity
Lips
Teeth

Tongue
Sublingual gland
Submandibular gland

Diaphragm
Liver
Cystic duct
Gallbladder

Duodenum

Ascending colon

Ileum

Cecum

Vermiform appendix

Parotid gland
Pharynx

Esophagus

Stomach
Hepatic duct
Pylorus
Pancreas
Transverse colon
Jejunum

Descending colon

Sigmoid colon

Rectum
Anus

Figure 6
Digestive System

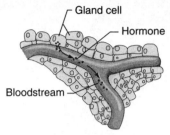

Gland cell

Hormone

Bloodstream

Endocrine gland
(ductless)

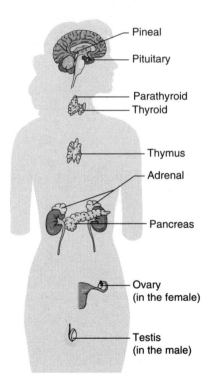

Pineal

Pituitary

Parathyroid
Thyroid

Thymus

Adrenal

Pancreas

Ovary
(in the female)

Testis
(in the male)

Figure 7
Endocrine System

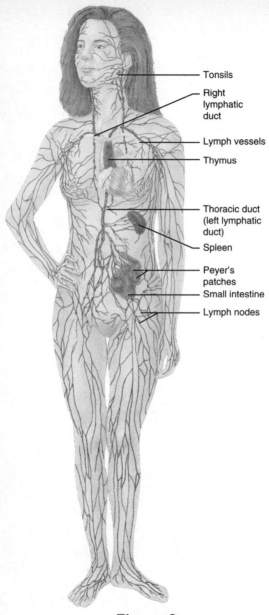

Tonsils

Right lymphatic duct

Lymph vessels

Thymus

Thoracic duct (left lymphatic duct)

Spleen

Peyer's patches

Small intestine

Lymph nodes

**Figure 8
Lymphatic System**

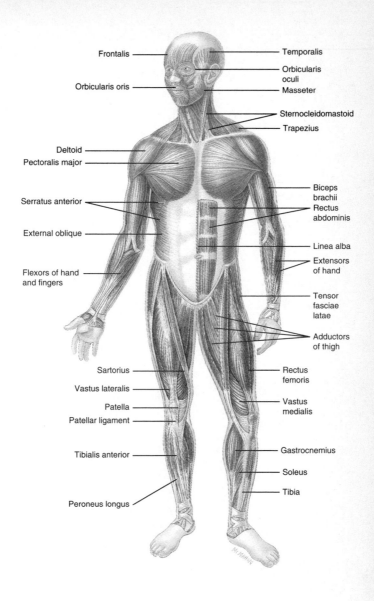

Frontalis — Temporalis

Orbicularis oculi

Orbicularis oris — Masseter

Sternocleidomastoid

Trapezius

Deltoid

Pectoralis major

Biceps brachii

Serratus anterior — Rectus abdominis

External oblique

Linea alba

Extensors of hand

Flexors of hand and fingers

Tensor fasciae latae

Adductors of thigh

Sartorius — Rectus femoris

Vastus lateralis

Patella

Patellar ligament — Vastus medialis

Tibialis anterior — Gastrocnemius

Soleus

Tibia

Peroneus longus

Figure 9
Muscles (Anterior)

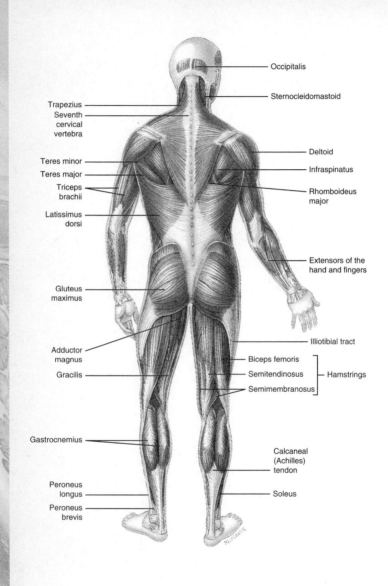

Occipitalis

Sternocleidomastoid

Trapezius

Seventh
cervical
vertebra

Deltoid

Teres minor

Infraspinatus

Teres major

Rhomboideus
major

Triceps
brachii

Latissimus
dorsi

Extensors of the
hand and fingers

Gluteus
maximus

Illiotibial tract

Adductor
magnus

Biceps femoris

Semitendinosus

Hamstrings

Gracilis

Semimembranosus

Gastrocnemius

Calcaneal
(Achilles)
tendon

Peroneus
longus

Soleus

Peroneus
brevis

Figure 10
Muscles (Posterior)

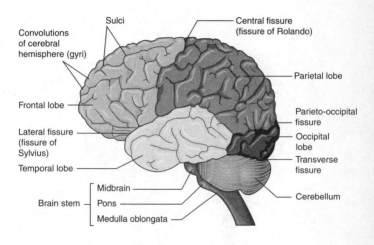

Lateral View of the Brain

Figure 11
Nervous System (Brain)

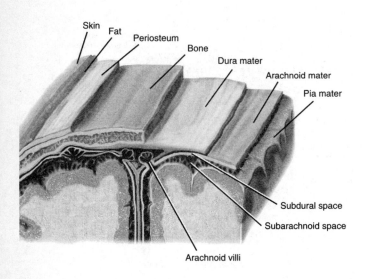

Figure 12
Nervous System (Meninges)

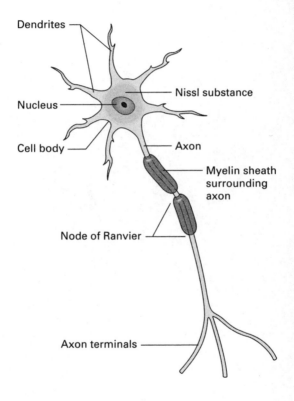

Figure 13
Nervous System (Bipolar Neuron)

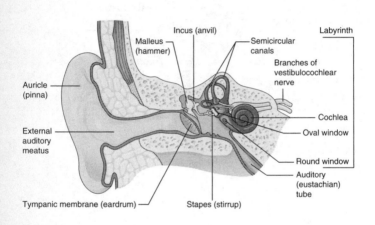

**Figure 14
Organs of Special Sense (Ear)**

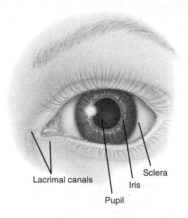

Lacrimal canals

Sclera

Iris

Pupil

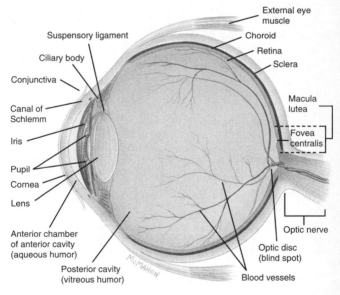

External eye muscle

Suspensory ligament

Choroid

Ciliary body

Retina

Conjunctiva

Sclera

Canal of Schlemm

Macula lutea

Iris

Fovea centralis

Pupil

Cornea

Lens

Anterior chamber of anterior cavity (aqueous humor)

Optic nerve

Posterior cavity (vitreous humor)

Optic disc (blind spot)

Blood vessels

Figure 15
Organs of Special Sense (Eye)

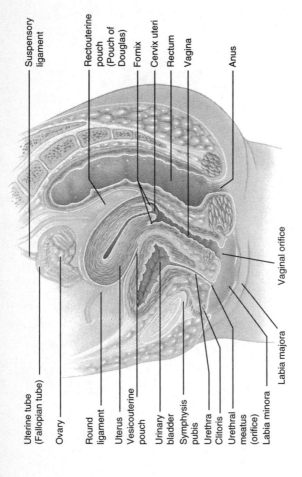

Uterine tube
(Fallopian tube)

Ovary

Round
ligament

Uterus

Vesicouterine
pouch

Urinary
bladder

Symphysis
pubis

Urethra

Clitoris

Urethral
meatus
(orifice)

Labia minora

Labia majora

Vaginal orifice

Suspensory
ligament

Rectouterine
pouch
(Pouch of
Douglas)

Fornix

Cervix uteri

Rectum

Vagina

Anus

**Figure 16
Reproductive System (Female)**

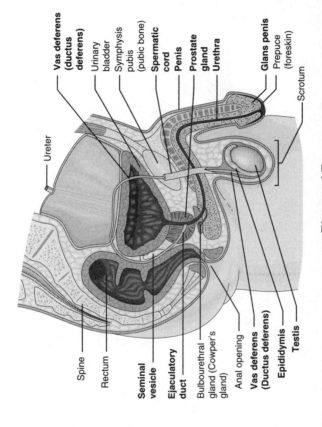

Figure 17
Reproductive System (Male)

Vas deferens (ductus deferens)
Urinary bladder
Symphysis pubis (pubic bone)
Spermatic cord
Penis
Prostate gland
Urethra
Glans penis
Prepuce (foreskin)
Scrotum

Ureter

Spine
Rectum
Seminal vesicle
Ejaculatory duct
Bulbourethral gland (Cowper's gland)
Anal opening
Vas deferens (Ductus deferens)
Epididymis
Testis

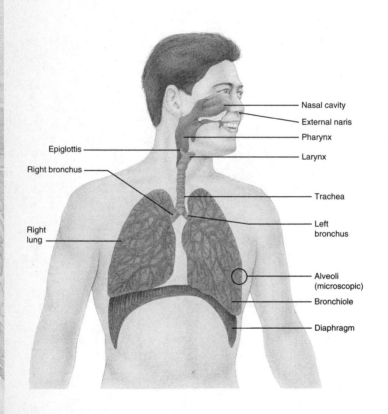

Nasal cavity

External naris

Pharynx

Epiglottis

Larynx

Right bronchus

Trachea

Right lung

Left bronchus

Alveoli (microscopic)

Bronchiole

Diaphragm

Figure 18
Respiratory System

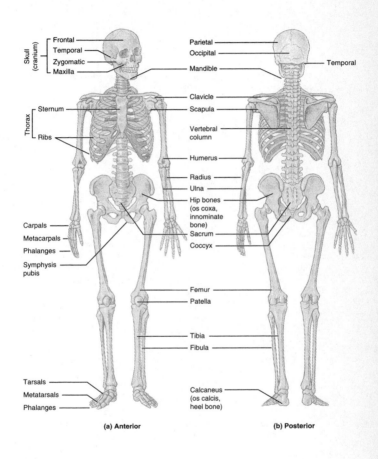

(a) Anterior

(b) Posterior

Figure 19
Skeletal System (Bones of the Body)

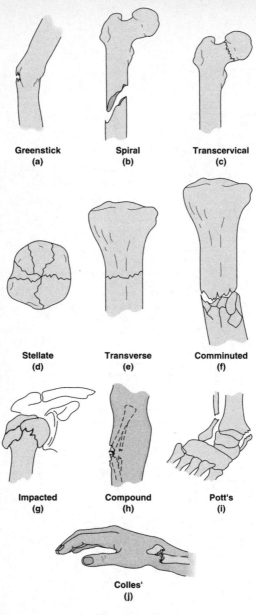

**Figure 20
Skeletal System (Fractures)**

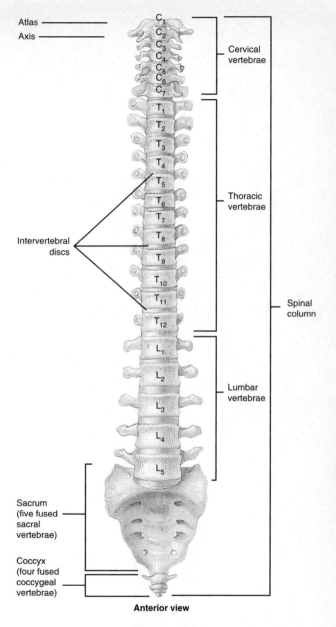

Atlas

Axis

Cervical
vertebrae

Thoracic
vertebrae

Intervertebral
discs

Spinal
column

Lumbar
vertebrae

Sacrum
(five fused
sacral
vertebrae)

Coccyx
(four fused
coccygeal
vertebrae)

C1
C2
C3
C4
C5
C6
C7
T1
T2
T3
T4
T5
T6
T7
T8
T9
T10
T11
T12
L1
L2
L3
L4
L5

Anterior view

Figure 21
Skeletal System (Vertebrae)

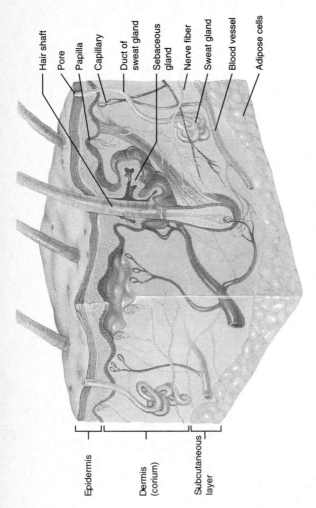

Hair shaft
Pore
Papilla
Capillary
Duct of sweat gland
Sebaceous gland
Nerve fiber
Sweat gland
Blood vessel
Adipose cells

Epidermis
Dermis (corium)
Subcutaneous layer

Figure 22
Skin

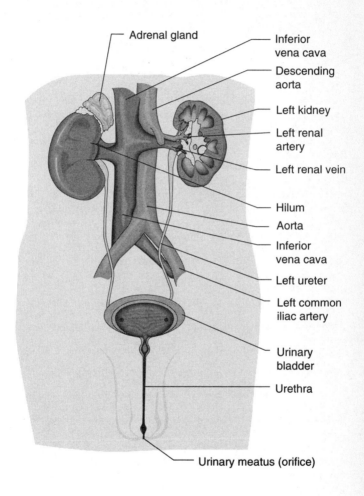

Adrenal gland

Inferior vena cava

Descending aorta

Left kidney

Left renal artery

Left renal vein

Hilum

Aorta

Inferior vena cava

Left ureter

Left common iliac artery

Urinary bladder

Urethra

Urinary meatus (orifice)

Figure 23
Urinary System

INDEX TO LABELED STRUCTURES FOUND IN FIGURES

Following is an index to the labeled structures appearing in the illustrations of the body systems. Use this index to conveniently find the anatomical structure of your choice.